PRAISE FOR *BEYOND MEDICINE*

"The principles and applications shared throughout this book will have your mind spinning with ideas that can transform your ministry or institution. You won't find every answer, but you will find many that can prevent you from 'reinventing the wheel' as you respond to the issues calling beyond the sick bed. Every medical missionary will find this book helpful enough to guarantee its place in their luggage as they go to serve."

Susan Carter, RN, MPH
Director Center for Medical Missions

"As a new missionary physician, the breadth of responsibilities I've faced has been daunting and at times overwhelming. As these challenges have arisen, I have gone to Dr. Stevens' material over and over, and have consistently found it to be intensely practical and helpful. All medical missionaries should have a copy of this book, and should refer to it often!"

Doug Lindberg, MD
Medical Missionary to Nepal

"David Stevens' book *Beyond Medicine* is a unique and priceless resource that should be on the desk of anyone currently involved in medical missions or planning to be, and within easy reach. I know that it will be on my desk and that I will be referring to it often. Every page shines with gems from David's considerable experience as a missionary doctor, hospital administrator, and CEO of CMDA. Again and again as I read I thought to myself, 'How I wish I'd known this 25 years ago!'"

David Thompson, MD
PAACS Director for Africa

PRAISE FOR *BEYOND MEDICINE*

"Practical, concise, relevant, wisdom born of experience, pearls on every page! My only regret is that this wonderful manual wasn't available twenty-five years ago. Thanks, David, for tackling the 'everything else' issues in medical missions!"

Dr. Bill McCoy
Medical Missionary

"Dr. David Stevens has drawn from his stellar track record as a medical missionary in Africa and an effective leader at home to address this crucial problem: healthcare missionaries are highly trained in medicine but totally unprepared for the many non-medical challenges they face in the developing world. *Beyond Medicine* fills that void. He moves from the operating room to the boardroom to the living room, telling a wealth of memorable stories of organizational dynamics, leadership, conflict, ethical dilemmas, and personal and family matters. While written for healthcare personnel, this book will have a wide application for any missionary who ends up in a totally unexpected leadership role! Where was this book when I needed it a generation ago?"

Neil O. Thompson, MD, FACS
Medical Mission Advocate

Christian Medical & Dental Associations®
Changing Hearts in Healthcare

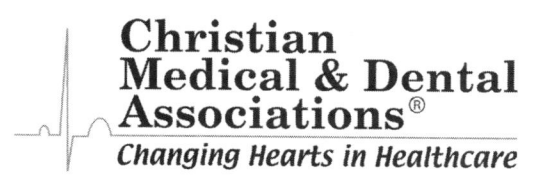

BEYOND MEDICINE

What Else You Need to Know to Be a Healthcare Missionary

David Stevens, MD, MA (Ethics)

Christian Medical & Dental Associations
P.O. Box 7500
Bristol, TN 37621
World Wide Web: www.cmda.org
E-mail: main@cmda.org

©2012 by Dr. David Stevens and Christian Medical & Dental Associations. All rights reserved. No part of this publication may be reproduced in any form without written permission from Christian Medical & Dental Associations.

Cover photo by Paul H. Stevens

Unless otherwise identified, all Scripture quotations are taken from the Holy Bible, New International Version®, Copyright© 1973, 1978, 1984, Biblica. Used by permission of Zondervan. All rights reserved.

ISBN 978-0-9706631-9-1
2012947619

Printed in the United States of America

In memory of Dr. Ernie Steury, humble missionary physician, founder of Tenwek Hospital, and my mentor.
Much of what I know, he taught me.

And to my dad Reverend Maurice Stevens, who modeled to me a hunger to share the gospel, a love for people, a boldness to step out in faith, and a willingness to serve to the ends of the earth.
I can't wait to hug you again in heaven.

ACKNOWLEDGEMENTS

As Solomon said, "...there is nothing new under the sun" (Ecclesiastes 1:9, NIV 1984). That is especially true when you write an instructional book. I've collected my knowledge from many people, filtered it from the perspective of the needs and challenges of healthcare missions, applied it, and learned from experience. I owe much to those who have taught and mentored me.

From my dad Reverend Maurice Stevens, a wonderful evangelist and people person, I learned public speaking and interpersonal skills. My mother, a teacher and great organizer, fostered discipline and a hunger for new knowledge. The basics of management and administration, I owe to the speakers at Christian Medical & Dental Associations' Continuing Medical and Dental Education conference held each year in Africa or Asia. Dr. Ernie Steury, my mentor as a young missionary, modeled how to apply important principles and gave me opportunities to gain experience young in my career. Little did I anticipate that I would be in charge of a 250-bed hospital five years out of residency!

World Gospel Mission, with whom we served, provided good orientation, great media training, and much more along my journey. Dr. David Kilel taught me how to integrate evangelism with healthcare and inspired me as he led thousands to Christ each year. Dr. Bob Andringa instilled a love for great governance as a foundation for successful ministry. Dr. Gene Rudd, my best friend and in reality my "co-CEO" at CMDA, has been my iron sharpening iron. We are both much better at what we do because of our close relationship.

I should acknowledge my staff at CMDA, an extraordinary group of leaders who are passionate about ministry. They have taught me as much as I have taught them. Two in particular had a profound impact on this book. Mandi Mooney, the editor of *Today's Christian Doctor*, compiled a diverse group of my writings into this volume, edited my scribbles, and oversaw this book's production. Thank you, Mandi! I couldn't have done this without you.

Susan Carter, the director of CMDA's Center of Medical Missions, has been our close family friend for more than thirty years. She served as a fellow missionary with us at Tenwek Hospital where we worked closely together to start a very successful community health program that radically changed peoples' lifestyles. That program was our laboratory to try all sorts of motivational, management, administrative and logistical techniques that were ultimately exported back to the hospital. After I left Tenwek, Susan was the hospital CEO and did a terrific job.

She challenged me to write a monthly column for the *e-Pistle*, a monthly resource distributed to CMDA's missionary members. Those articles are the foundation of this book. Susan, this book would not exist without you! Thanks for putting up with me in those early days when what I knew and practiced was much less than now!

I also want to acknowledge my wife Jody. You were my faithful companion and confidant during medical school and residency, through eleven years of missionary service in Kenya, to sending me off to war zones to do relief ministry while we served with Samaritan's Purse, and then finally saw how God could use me to lead CMDA long before I did. You are the love of my life!

Most of all I want to thank my Lord and Savior Jesus Christ who said, "Follow me, and I will make you fisher's of men" (Matthew 4:19, ESV). Little did I understand as a senior in high school what an incredible journey that would be and the important lessons He would teach me along the way.

To Him be all the glory!

TABLE OF CONTENTS

Introduction   10

Part 1: Leadership Skills
1. Leadership   14
2. Motivating People to Change   32
3. Communication Essentials   40
4. Presenting a Heart-Changing Message   48
5. Ignore the Grapevine and It Will Hang You   56

Part 2: Ethics
6. Medical Mission Bioethics   64
7. Short-Term Ethics   72
8. The Noble Pursuit of Medicine   76

Part 3: Planning and Administration
9. Boards That Work   90
10. The CEO   100
11. Senior Staff   106
12. Mid-Level Managers   112
13. Strategic Planning   120

Part 4: Organizational Monitoring
14. Developing the Christian Workplace   138
15. Situational Analysis   146
16. Eminent or Preeminent   150
17. The Art of Running a Meeting   154

Part 5: Budgets and Finances
18. Budgeting and the Missionary Doctor   162
19. Dissociative Thinking   166

Part 6: Personnel Matters
    20. Your Most Needed Resource   172
    21. Conflict Resolution   178
    22. Orienting Short-Term Medical Missionaries   190
    23. Basic Training   194
    24. Oiling the Gears   196
    25. To Catch a Thief   202

Part 7: Missional Situations
    26. Spiritual Ministry in Medical Missions   210
    27. Medical Missions STAT!   216
    28. Perfecting Your Prayer Letter   226
    29. Raising Big Bucks   232

Part 8: Community Projects
    30. Turbocharging Community Health   240
    31. Train Up   264

Part 9: Family Focus
    32. Family Matters   276
    33. School Daze   282

Part 10: Personal Areas
    34. Self-Care   290
    35. Forgiveness   294
    36. Flameout   298
    37. Points on Time   302
    38. Cachinnation   308
    39. Leaving Without Leaving   312
    40. Wealth Management   316

Final Thoughts   320

Appendix   325

Photo Gallery   335

INTRODUCTION

I went to a great medical school and an outstanding family practice residency program. I thought I was well-trained, and I was certainly eager to get to the overseas mission field to "save lives and stamp out disease" with a large portion of evangelism on the side. "Get ready Africa, here I come!"

Like most new missionaries, I was a little apprehensive about all the new diseases I would have to diagnose and treat, the large number of patients I would need to see each day, and the lack of support staff, supplies, and diagnostic capabilities. All the same, I wasn't fearful because, like most healthcare professionals, I wasn't afraid to work hard. Studying medicine had made me a fast learner, plus older missionaries were available for questions. If they had learned to function well without all the things we enjoy in Western healthcare, I could too.

Still, the first year was like doing my internship again. I learned to use fishing line for retention sutures, utilize amnion for a burn dressing, treat neonatal tetanus, see that constipation was the cardinal sign of amebiasis in our area of Kenya, and thousands of other things. Despite the challenges, it was intellectually stimulating and fulfilling to make a dramatic difference in so many patients' lives and see dozens of them come to the Lord each day. There was definitely a steep learning curve, but it wasn't an impossible one. In fact, I loved expanding my "scope of practice" and soon realized that medical missionaries have some of the broadest levels of experience of any doctors in the world.

What I didn't realize initially was that learning to practice medicine overseas was the easy part. I was trained to continually learn about medicine over my lifetime so that came naturally. The hard part was handling all the non-medical responsibilities thrust upon me.

I wasn't the only one. You hear all the time about healthcare professionals saying, "If I could just practice medicine then…." In the U.S., they say it because of the huge increase in bureaucracy and the hassles of dealing with third party payers. On the mission field, you hear it because you have to do so many things that you weren't trained to do—like governance, management, administration, recruitment, staff discipline, financial supervision, donor relations, security oversight, strategic planning, spiritual ministry, project administration, fundraising, government and church relations, community health, development, and the list goes on. If you are already overseas, I don't need to convince you. If you are still preparing, you probably won't have to do everything on that list, but I assure you that you will have to do many things that no one trained you to do.

Even more, the overall success of your ministry will depend more on your abilities to do non-medical tasks than on the fact that you are a great nurse, pharmacist, or physician. These other duties keep the ship of your outreach heading in the right direction, but also ensure its integrity during storms of adversity and its readiness in calm seas to take advantage of opportunities.

This book originated as a decade of articles I wrote for *The e-Pistle*, a monthly resource of the Christian Medical & Dental Association's Center for Medical Missions. It is circulated to more than 1,300 medical missionaries around the world. The articles are based on my eleven years of experience as a missionary doctor in Kenya providing leadership at Tenwek Hospital, as well as my work as the Director of World Medical Missions where I visited mission health programs around the world and gained insights from each one. I also owe a special debt of gratitude to the pioneer missionary, Dr. Ernie Steury, who had twenty-two years of know-how before he began to mentor me.

I trust this book will inspire you to be the leader you need to be. I desire that it will not only educate you but also encourage you to become a lifelong student of the important topics it introduces. I hope its wealth of practical suggestions will give you the tools you need to carry out your call well in service to the Lord. If so, my prayers have been answered.

David Stevens, MD, MA (Ethics)
CEO, Christian Medical & Dental Associations

PART 1
LEADERSHIP SKILLS

CHAPTER 1
LEADERSHIP

Harry S. Truman once said, "Progress occurs when courageous, skillful leaders seize the opportunity to change things for the better." In successful organizations, it boils down to leadership. It is the fuel for success and progress whether you are President of the United States or a physician, nurse, or other member of the staff in a medical mission outreach. Unfortunately, the most overlooked skill necessary for success in missionary medicine is leadership. It's a skill that is not taught in medical or dental school; yet, almost every missionary doctor is required to lead in some way. Some do a great job, others muddle through, and many fall short.

Some people are natural leaders, but more often leadership is a skill learned like any other. In fact, the Bible is full of stories of God looking for and training reluctant leaders, from Joshua to Moses and Peter to Esther. We read in 1 Samuel 13:14 of God's search for David, "...the Lord has sought out a man after his own heart and appointed him leader of his people..." (NIV 1984). He also searched for a leader for the Israelites in Ezekiel 22:30, "I looked for a man among them who would build up the wall and stand before me in the gap on behalf of the land so I would not have to destroy it..." (NIV 1984). The world is in desperate need of godly leaders, and God continues to look for those who will stand in the gap.

So what is leadership? The dictionary has it wrong. It states that a leader is "somebody who guides or directs others by showing them the way or telling them how to behave or the head of an organization such as a nation, political party, or military." These definitions confuse the power someone has over others or the position they hold with true leadership.

In its most basic sense, leadership means the ability to influence others to change. Leaders figure out where the group needs to go and what will help them get there. It is not the power to force others to their way of doing things.

It is also easy to confuse being a leader with being a manager. People want a manager when life is orderly, predictable, and things are going well. Managers tweak the system that already exists to make it better without causing major disruption or emotional consequences. They exercise the power of their position. True leaders bring change and people want them when change is needed because things are unpredictable, uncomfortable, or even out of control. Neville Chamberlin, Prime Minister of Great Britain, was a good manager but a woeful leader when World War II was about to break out. He hung onto the status quo at all costs, including appeasing Germany. War broke out and who did the people call to provide leadership? Winston Churchill. He was a true leader who led England to victory through a myriad of changes and seemingly unbearable hardship.

Biblically, is it right to have the ambition to be a leader? Doesn't Jeremiah 45:5 say, "Should you then seek great things for yourself? Seek them not?" (NIV 1984). But turn to 1 Timothy 3:1 and read, "To aspire to leadership is an honorable ambition" (NEB).

To reconcile these two verses, you need to understand there are two types of ambition. Jeremiah is referring to having the ambition for power and prestige. In Latin, the word he uses for "ambition" means, "campaigning for yourself" and that is not biblical. Paul talks about a different type of ambition for leadership. An ambition to servant leadership as Christ defined it in Mark 10:43-44, "...whoever wants to become great among you must be your servant, and whoever wants to be first must be slave of all" (NIV 1984). Christ, the greatest leader and influencer who ever lived, demonstrated that kind of leadership. As someone said, "Because the children of Adam want to become great He became small. Because we will not stoop, He humbled Himself. Because we want to rule, He came to serve."

Throughout history, true leaders have been in short supply. We read of how God searched for true servant leaders to partner with Him in building the kingdom. He found:

- David – "…the Lord has sought out a man after his own heart and appointed him leader of his people…" (1 Samuel 13:14, NIV 1984).
- Ezekiel – "I looked for a man among them who would build up the wall and stand before me in the gap on behalf of the land so I would not have to destroy it…" (Ezekiel 22:30, NIV 1984).
- Paul – "…I have appeared to you to appoint you as a servant and as a witness of what you have seen of me…" (Acts 26:16, NIV 1984).

Some people are natural leaders. Look at the life of Joseph, for example. Wherever he went, he led—in Potiphar's house, in prison, and before Pharaoh. Not all natural leaders are good leaders though. Look at the charisma of Adolf Hitler who influenced millions to evil. For your missionary service to be successful, you need to lead patients to change their health habits and staff to change their work habits. You will need to lead in your mission, workplace, family, and community.

The good news is that leadership skills can be nurtured. I think I was born with some natural leadership ability, but it was strengthened by leadership training, mentoring, and working with humble servant leaders who were my role models. Let me share with you some of what I learned to reveal key attributes of a good leader.

Vision
Good leaders have vision. They are dissatisfied with the status quo. This is what drives their desire to lead change. I constantly remind my staff that "there is a better way to do everything and we are out to find it." I reiterate that change will be required in order to accomplish this.

A true leader has a vision of where the people or organization he or she leads needs to go. A leader understands the mission and, as they say in industry, "Defines the business of our business." They not only have a vision but also can articulate it. Vision is the ability to set the trail for others to follow. That is why the best test of whether someone is a true leader is to look and see if anyone is following.

Strategy
The second characteristic of a leader is someone who is a strategizer.

It is not enough to just have vision. If so, you are a dreamer of no practical consequence. A good leader knows where you need to go and also has a map they will share to show you how to get there. A strategy that is worthy to follow also must be doable. That doesn't equate with easy. Change is often difficult and the bigger the vision, the more complex and time consuming the strategy that may have to be employed.

I've found the best way to do the "impossible" is to develop my strategy by working backward from the ultimate goal. Instead of asking myself what I should do first, I ask what is the last thing I need to accomplish to reach my goal. Then, I identify the precursor to that until I get back to the first thing I need to do.

If I were a leader in a U.S. office practice, my vision might be for every patient to feel they have been taken care of by the Great Physician. To reach that goal, each patient needs to feel loved and have their medical, spiritual, and emotional needs met. To accomplish this, how do I make patients feel loved? I need the right atmosphere, good communication, timeliness, and a caring staff. To create the right atmosphere, I take out the TV, create a comfortable homey waiting area, add helpful Christian magazines, put on soft instrumental Christian music, place some inspiring art on the walls, and make sure each patient is welcomed into our office "home." I make sure each person is greeted personally. I do away with the sliding glass window which was a barrier between my staff and patients and put my receptionist at a desk in the waiting area. She stands up and greets every patient and their family as they enter, and asks them to sit down at her desk to get information. I then serve coffee and tea. Once you have a clear goal, you can work backward to figure out how to reach it.

John Mott, the founder of the YMCA and one of the launchers of the modern Protestant mission movement, summed it up this way, "A leader is a man who knows the road, can keep ahead, and who pulls others after him."

Motivation
A good leader must learn how to motivate people to embrace change or as Mott said, to "pull others after." Persuasive communication is an art that can be learned. It starts first by understanding where peo-

ple are so you can reach back to them. Secondly, you need to realize what already mobilizes them to embrace change, and then thirdly, to link the changes you propose to those motivation switches. In the early days of his startup company, the founder of Apple Steve Jobs was trying to recruit a top Coca-Cola executive to his team. He realized that a prime motivator for this man was investing his life where it would make a difference, so he sent him a note saying, "Do you want to make sugar water for the rest of your life, or do you want to change the world?" The man moved to Apple.

Good leaders have strong convictions and are not hesitant to convey them to others. They share their vision with confidence, which is important and thus worth being committed to.

Good leaders motivate others to accept a vision and commit to making it happen. Admiral Chester Nimitz, the great World War II Navy leader said, "Leadership may be defined as that quality that inspires sufficient confidence in subordinates so they are willing to accept his views and carry out his commands." Someone else took leadership to another level when they said, "A good leader inspires men to have confidence in him; a great leader inspires them to have confidence in themselves."

Good motivators also understand human nature. Everyone wants to be recognized and rewarded for their accomplishments. Everyone wants to be respected, to be listened to, and to apply their skills toward something that makes a difference. Link these and other universal motivators to what you want to accomplish and you will motivate people. This helps create a psychological bond between you and those you lead, allowing you to: inspire confidence in people who are frightened; catalyze action where there is hesitation; instill strength where there is weakness; and give hope that the future will be better.

Empathy
Good leaders are empathetic. Work on developing empathy, an ability to get into others' heads to understand their needs and motivators. Continually ask questions to understand those needs. Then connect your communication to the needs and motivators that you have identified to get people to accept change. When I speak on physician-assisted suicide (PAS), I tell people that it is dangerous for physicians,

patients, and their families. That does not make my point nearly as well as illustrating a key point with an empathetic story.

Can you imagine going to visit your mother in the nursing home one morning and finding her bed empty? You ask the nurse where she is and she replies, "Didn't they tell you? She asked her doctor for a lethal prescription and she committed suicide last night." How would you feel? I would be asking myself, "Why didn't she say something? Did she think we didn't love her? Did we not visit her often enough? Was she afraid that we don't want to be burdened with the cost of her care? Did the doctor influence her to do this?" There are many more victims of suicide than the one who died. If we legalize PAS, this could happen to you.

Empathy puts you into someone else's shoes and you see the issue from their point of view, their concerns, and their priorities.

President Harry S. Truman, a student of good leadership principles, emphasized the leader's role in motivation with this tongue-in-cheek comment, "A leader is someone who can get others to do what they don't want to do and like it!"

Cherished Values
Not only is a good leader a good motivator with strong convictions and empathy, they also communicate a strong set of values that says, "This is who we are and this is how we act." I expect my CMDA staff to treat every member like they would want to be treated. When you call, you do not want to be referred from person to person without your problem being resolved or your question being answered. You want someone to go to bat for you and get the information you need. I want every one of my employees to handle each member contact like they are dealing with their own family member or best friend and go out of their way to solve the problem.

Wise Recruiter
An excellent leader realizes that they cannot accomplish their mission alone. They need to recruit the right kind of people to work with them. The best measurement of a leader is to see the kind of person that is attracted to follow them.

I look at the Five C's when I evaluate prospective employees:

- Christian Commitment – Does this person really know Christ as their Savior and is their life different because of it? Do they exercise spiritual disciplines?
- Character – Is this a person of integrity and have they demonstrated it in their life in their honesty, work ethic, relationships, etc.?
- Chemistry – How will this person fit in with my present team? Will they blend in and work well? Will others value their contributions and get along with them? Are they going to be sand or oil in the organizational gears?
- Competency – Does this person have the skills and experience to accomplish what I am hiring them to do? Are they a self-starter and a problem solver or am I going to have to look over their shoulder all the time? Are they teachable?
- Calling – After learning as much about our organization and getting to know our key personnel, does this person sense a calling from God to join our ministry? Do we sense God's direction to make this person part of our CMDA family?

A good leader finds people who are smarter than he or she is in their area of expertise and then helps them find fulfillment in their role by helping them to be all that God designed them to be.

A Psychological Bond

Great leaders like Winston Churchill inspire their followers to be better. They establish a deep psychological bond. They help their followers have confidence when they are frightened and certainty when they are vacillating. Remember Churchill's words after the successful Normandy invasion when some were vacillating and encouraging Britain to sue for peace? He said, "Now this is not the end. It is not even the beginning of the end, but it is, perhaps, the end of the beginning."

Great leaders move people to action when there is inaction. America was very reluctant to get involved in World War II. Many in Washington didn't want to even provide armaments to England, which was being bombed and increasingly cut off from the sea by German U-boat attacks. To move the U.S. from inaction to action, Churchill said in a radio speech, "Here is the answer which I will give to President Roosevelt...We shall not fail or falter; we shall not weaken or tire. Neither the sudden shock of battle nor the long-drawn trials of vigilance and exertion will wear us down. Give us the tools and we will finish the job."

A good leader inspires strength where there is weakness. When they were reeling from the retreat at Dunkirk and the prospect of Germany invading across the English Channel, Churchill said to his countrymen, "Never give in—never, never, never, never, in nothing great or small, large or petty, never give in except to convictions of honor and good sense. Never yield to force; never yield to the apparently overwhelming might of the enemy."

He also instilled courage that banished cowardice. He said, "One ought never to turn one's back on a threatened danger and try to run away from it. If you do that, you will double the danger. But if you meet it promptly and without flinching, you will reduce the danger by half." And then before the British Parliament in a speech just after Dunkirk on June 4, 1940, "We shall fight on the beaches, we shall fight on the landing grounds, we shall fight in the fields and in the streets, we shall fight in the hills; we shall never surrender…."

Great leaders instill optimism where there is cynicism. Churchill again, "Let us therefore brace ourselves to our duty, and so bear ourselves that if the British Empire and its Commonwealth last for a thousand years, men will still say, This was their finest hour." A pessimist sees the difficulty in every opportunity; an optimist sees the opportunity in ever difficulty. Does the psychological bond you share with your team members inspire them to greatness?

Problem Solver
I tell my senior staff that if we did not have problems, we would not have jobs. A competent leader has to timely solve problems and resolve conflicts. Managers often ignore small problems until they become big ones, as if they will simply go away by ignoring them. Or instead of dealing with a relationship issue or a specific problem employee, they make a new policy. That can bring everyone down to the lowest common denominator and restrict everyone's creativity and joy.

Here are some principles to help you be a better problem solver:

- Deal with small problems before they become big problems.
- Take the time to understand the issue from all significant points of view.
- Determine your options for solving the problem.
- Seek advice from wise counselors if the best option is not clear.
- Make a decision and implement it.
- Timely reevaluate how the solution is working. Is the problem solved?
- Recycle the process until the issue is resolved.

A few more Churchillisms? "Kites rise highest against the wind, not with it." "Difficulties mastered are opportunities won."

<u>Exemplary</u>
Character counts, especially in leadership. A leader needs to be respected and trusted. You cannot influence people without these two exemplary characteristics. That means you are a person of integrity. Read these verses.

- "Now the overseer must be above reproach, the husband of but one wife, temperate, self-controlled, respectable, hospitable, able to teach" (1 Timothy 3:2, NIV 1984).
- "Since an overseer is entrusted with God's work, he must be blameless—not overbearing, not quick-tempered, not given to drunkenness, not violent, not pursuing dishonest gain" (Titus 1:7, NIV 1984).

People will not follow someone they do not respect and admire. Focus on developing good character and showing integrity in every situation. Strive to become more Christ-like, to become more like the greatest leader who ever lived.

Your followers may not agree with every decision you make, but they are confident you are endeavoring to act biblically, in their best interest, and in the best interest of the organization. They are confident you are fair, truthful, and honorable. You are willing to admit your mistakes and take responsibility for them. As one person said, "A real leader faces the music even when he dislikes the tune."

Good leaders need to be organized. It takes organization to move a group forward. So work on developing your organizational skills, or surround yourself with people who are organized and can fill in for this deficiency. How you attend to phone calls and e-mails, keep appointments, and accomplish tasks can either enhance or damage your influence and reputation.

One of the most exemplary traits of great leaders is accountability. They are not only afraid of outside scrutiny, they welcome it. They respect those they are responsible to and are transparent with them.

Stewardship of People
Great leaders see their people as a sacred trust. I have seen so-called leaders who use people like some people use Kleenex. They rule by intimidation and fear or alternate that with largess. An employee cannot tell if they are going to get emotionally hugged or strangled at any given time. They operate like an abusive husband or parent, destroying individual confidence and abusing their position of authority. Employees finally flee but are often permanently damaged. Others in positions of power are not cruel or abusive, but their employees are seen as units of production valued for what they accomplish, not who they are.

God has a different standard of leadership. God's word teaches that we have a spiritual responsibility for those we lead or supervise. We should help people develop and become all God designed them to be. As leaders, our task is to help those we lead to develop their spiritual gifts and competency skills, and to grow emotionally, socially, and in every aspect of life.

In the midst of projects and deadlines, I try to remind myself it is more important to develop people than new resources or programs. Invest your time and efforts in building people. Be available to help with personal issues and to make sure your staff's skills are expanding and growing. If you really care about the individuals you lead, these things will flow naturally with Christ as our example. His relationship with His "staff" of twelve men is our model. He taught, challenged, and exemplified to them what it means to be a true God follower.

To help those you lead be successful, you need to provide them with continuing training to increase their knowledge, the tools they need to equip them to be successful, and the right level of delegation to stretch but not over challenge them. You need to adequately compensate them, provide opportunities for feedback, and hold them accountable.

Willing
Good leaders are willing to:

- Be Scrutinized – As a leader, you will be put under the microscope with a resultant loss of privacy and anonymity. Your actions, words, and writing will be evaluated to figure out what you "really were trying to say or do." A high level of scrutiny goes hand-in-hand with leadership.

- Pay the Price – Providing great leadership is hard work. Leaders must also be willing to pay the price it costs in time and energy to stay in front of the group. Good leaders don't expect anyone to work harder than they do. You need to lead from the front, not just by saying what the standard is but in going above and beyond it in your words and actions. I make a point of helping to clean up after a CMDA party function, do my own dishes at lunch, contribute more than my share, and work longer hours than most of my staff. (I've got a couple of workaholics that I'm more than happy to award with the "hardest worker prize!") When I was a missionary doctor, I made a statement when I picked up the extra call or covered a ward that was short staffed.

- Take a Punch – Leaders need to have a healthy self-confidence. Leaders will be criticized, misunderstood, and even ridiculed. Churchill was. He said, "You have enemies? Good. That means you've stood up for something, sometime in your life." Are you willing to take the punches? Someone once said, "If you're not afraid to face the music, you may someday lead the band." Staying focused on your vision and goals helps deflect the punches that come to all those who step out in front of the crowd.

    Hardly a day goes by that I do not get criticism from someone. (It is impossible to please all doctors, all the time!) I make a habit of listening to criticism and honestly asking myself if it is merited or constructive. If so, I learn and change from it. Sometimes though, the criticism needs to flow off my back like water off a duck's back while I still show grace and love to those who criticize me. My standard is to respond personally to each criticism that comes from a legitimate source. This sometimes opens an opportunity for incredible ministry because there may be another problem someone is dealing with and I just happened to be the target of opportunity when someone blew their stack.

I remember a neurosurgeon who called upset because he had been approached for a gift to our capital campaign. The criticism was directed at me but I was out of the office, so CMDA's Senior Vice President Dr. Gene Rudd spoke with him. With grace and sensitivity, he responded to the criticism. Before the phone call was over, he was praying with the doctor who was devastated from losing a patient on the table the night before and from a child who was no longer following the Lord. His anger expressed towards us was in reality a call for help.

- To Fail – Good leaders can handle failure and then try again. Fear of failure chokes leadership and incapacitates decision-making. It is inevitable that you will make some bad decisions, say something you should not have, or fire someone you hired. When you fail, learn from it, apologize if you need to, pick yourself up, dust yourself off, and get back in the race. Just don't make a habit of it! "Success is the ability to go from one failure to another with no loss of enthusiasm." My staff members know I expect them to fail sometimes. If not, they are probably not taking risks or going out on the limb of faith. Leaders need to learn how to deal with their own failures and help others profit from theirs.

- To Stick it Out - Great leaders are ordinary people with extraordinary determination. Look at Abraham Lincoln who failed in election after election before he finally became president. He is arguably the greatest leader to ever occupy the White House. No matter how big the failure on the battlefield or in Congress, he got up, brushed himself off, and kept going.

Though Dr. Ernie Steury was bone-tired after being the only doctor at Tenwek for ten years and people were encouraging him to quit, he stuck with it. He had a vision of a mission hospital meeting the needs of the Kipsigis people and bringing many to Christ. I'm guessing everyone will be tempted to quit at some point, but perseverance will undoubtedly lead to many wonderful surprises around the bend. In a real sense, sticking it out is not because of our determination but because of God's calling and the reality of His faithfulness. If we stand firm on that foundation, we cannot be moved.

- To Seek God's Will – The greatest pitfall for great leaders is their own pride and abilities. Great leaders become footnotes in history if they do not realize their own inadequacy and seek God's guidance. As someone said, "It is always wise to look ahead, but difficult to look further than you can see."

As you plan and make decisions, pray this verse, "Show me your ways, O Lord, teach me your paths" (Psalm 25:4, NIV 1984). To be a good guide, you must first follow the greatest leader.

Maintain Balance

One of the toughest tasks leaders face is balancing the multitude of demands placed on you from many different groups—your colleagues, employees, the community, family, friends, supervisors, the government, your mission, the local church, and the list goes on. For want of a better word, it takes wisdom, or what the world calls "political sense," to balance often conflicting demands for your time, energy, and presence. You need to set your priorities first. To hit the target of balance, you first have to determine what balance looks like.

Then you need to learn how to graciously say, "No." The more successful you are, the more people will want a "piece" of you. They will flatter your ego by telling you how indispensable you are and how large their need is that only you can fill. Much of our over-commitment comes from not taking the time to envision a life of equilibrium and then setting boundaries to protect it.

The keystone of maintaining balance is to keep the most important things the most important things. First, you must prioritize your relationship with God. You will not survive long in ministry without it and there is no standing still. You are either growing in Christ or moving further away from Him. Entropy naturally occurs unless you are proactive to fight against it. Second, you need to do only what you can do—have great relationships with your spouse and children if you have them. Third is your responsibility to serve God with your talents, efforts, and abilities in what He has called you to do.

One of the challenges I face is keeping the proper balance between developing and maintaining relationships and getting things done. I tend to err towards the latter. Some have the other problem. They spend so much time nurturing their relationships that they don't give their work the attention it needs. Finding homeostasis so that your life is healthy in all its aspects is a key to effective leadership.

Power Plays
Exceptional leaders know how to use their power rightly and effectively. There are four types of power:

- Positional Power – The authority you have over people because of your position. Taken to the extreme, exercising positional power ends up in dictatorship.
- Expert Power – The expertise and ability you have that others do not have to do a job. If you are the only surgeon, you have expert power in the surgical arena. Your expert power causes people to look to you for answers because of the knowledge and experience you have.
- Personal Attraction – Some individuals have power because of their charisma. People do what they say because they like them and do not want to displease them.
- Effort Power – You put forth a greater effort than others and are thus more dedicated to accomplishing the mission of the group you lead.

There is a time to use each of these types of power. The last three are the best to use but the first may be needed and you cannot step back when it is time for it to be applied. Just like children with good parents know, those you lead need to realize there are certain lines they cross at their peril. Cross those lines and they will experience predictable unpleasant consequences. Knowing that engenders respect and also causes people to stay in the boundaries. You do not have to exercise your positional power often if those you lead know where the fences are and that you will enforce them.

Several years ago, a staff member wrote an anonymous letter to another employee threatening him. Ridiculously, he accused him of surreptitiously supporting a denominational theological point of view in a chapel message that he did not agree with. He had crossed the boundary. I do not accept anonymously written letters threatening bodily harm. When I found out about it, I fired him on the spot.

A good leader knows how and when to use each of the four types of leadership power and does so effectively.

Spiritual Leadership
No matter how many of the above characteristics you manifest, you will not get far in good Christian organizations unless you manifest spiritual leadership as well. We've touched on a few of the traits of spiritual leadership, but let's summarize them here.

God assigns us to be leaders. There are lots of great examples of this in the Bible. There was Moses at the burning bush. God's selection of Joshua is recorded in Deuteronomy 31:14a, "The Lord said to Moses, 'Now the day of your death is near. Call Joshua and present yourselves at the Tent of Meeting, where I will commission him'"(NIV 1984). Christ called the disciples individually to follow Him. Paul had his Damascus road experience. When God told Ananias to go to Paul, He said, "Go! I have picked him as my personal representative to non-Jews and kings and Jews" (Acts 9:15, MSG).

God does His calling in many different ways, and each call is different. You may have a dramatic calling like Paul where God speaks to you in your mind through a Scripture, a message, or a song. Through this, you know He is giving you specific directions. Many missionaries can point to God's calling in this way. You may have someone like Moses who recognizes that God has equipped you for leadership. They may ask you to assume a leadership position in your church, ministry, or profession.

God may provide an opportunity for leadership. Perhaps there is a need for a leader, and as you go to God you have a growing realization that you should be that person. You may accept that direction with fear and trepidation in your heart. You may feel unprepared and unskilled for what God wants you to do. Think about that for a minute. What if Moses had said "No!" to God's call to go down to Egypt? It is clear that he wanted it to be anyone but him. God would still have accomplished His purpose without Moses, but then Moses would have been a footnote in history, at best. He wouldn't have had the blessing of seeing God working in or through him.

In this day and time, individuals are more reluctant than ever to be leaders. We see it on our campuses. No one wants to get out in front to pay the price or reap the blessings of leadership in their own lives. I have seen it in medical mission outreaches where the work suffers because those with the capabilities come up with excuses—I need to spend more time with my family, my workload is heavy already—to not step up. And the ministry flounders or limps along leaderless. The bottom line is not what you or I want, but what does God want? More than our skills and abilities, God wants our willingness.

The other spiritual principal of leadership is that suffering is often involved. Peter's words should resonate from 1 Peter 4:12, "Dear friends, do not be surprised at the painful trial you are suffering, as though something strange were happening to you" (NIV 1984). If you are a leader, you will bear burdens, endure the loneliness of making difficult decisions, have individuals disappoint and even betray you, have your dreams shattered, be criticized fairly and unfairly, and sometimes fail. If you try to lead in your own power, you will soon be discouraged.

If you depend on God and let His love shine through you in difficult times, you will be like a broken perfume bottle releasing the fragrance of God. You will experience a peace that passes all understanding. Through the Holy Spirit, you will find strength welling up in your soul as you seek God as it promises in Isaiah 40:31, "But they who wait upon the Lord will get new strength. They will rise up with wings like eagles. They will run and not get tired. They will walk and not become weak" (NLV). You will find His strength made perfect in your weakness. Suffering is a small price to pay to experience God working in and through you!

The Bible also teaches that if we are to be a good leader, we must first be a great servant. Matthew 23:11 states, "Do you want to stand out? Then step down. Be a servant" (MSG). The character of a servant leader is magnetic and magnetizing. Like rubbing a pin with a piece of silk, people want to get close to a servant leader to become magnetic themselves. People get a servant's heart as they come in contact with a real servant who becomes their role model and example. The longer I live, the more I realize that having a servant's heart is the key component to influence. 1 Timothy 3:13 points this out, "Those who do this servant work will come to be highly respected, a real credit to this Jesus-faith" (MSG).

Where does it come from? It comes out of a great love for God and a great love for people. It comes from realizing how limited you are and how unlimited God is. It comes from being filled with God's Holy Spirit. When you truly serve God, you can truly serve others.

Well, let me sum it up. Whether we realize it or not, we are all influencing someone or some group—our friends, our family, our church, our workplace. By learning some basic leadership principles and applying them to your life, you can become a much better leader and have incredible influence in others' lives.

Becoming a better leader boils down to just two things. Are you willing to lead and are you willing to learn?

True leaders make an enormous difference in the lives of others. One of my favorite stories is of Dr. John Geddie, a Presbyterian missionary from Scotland. In 1848, he went to the Samoan island of Aneityum. He found head hunters, cannibals, and terrible heathen practices. When a man died, his wife was immediately strangled to prevent her from being a burden on the society.

Dr. Geddie served God on this small isolated island for twenty-four years. By the time he retired, that small island of 3,500 inhabitants had a church that seated one thousand people! His incredible leadership and influence were inscribed in two sentences on his tombstone: "When he landed, there were no Christians. When he left, there were no heathen." What do you want your tombstone to say? I hope it is something like that!

CHAPTER 2
MOTIVATING PEOPLE TO CHANGE

How do you motivate people to change their behavior? I don't know about you, but that wasn't a topic they covered when I went to medical school. Oh, we had talks on the importance of patient education, but that missed the point. Knowledge is not the key to changing how people act.

Let's back up. Why is motivating people to change such an important skill for you to master? First, you need to influence your healthcare team—your colleagues and subordinate staff—to do their jobs better. What needs to improve around your hospital or clinic? My long list would include motivating staff to keep the hospital clean, show compassion, have spiritual ministry with each patient, and provide medicines and therapy on time.

You also need to motivate both your patients and your community to change their health practices. When I arrived at Tenwek in 1981, the hospital was averaging 185 percent occupancy with two, sometimes three patients to a bed. At one point during a malaria epidemic, we had 485 inpatients in our 135-bed hospital! Days and nights were long as we took care of a never-ending stream of patients. A look at our statistics revealed that preventable diseases were the cause of at least half of our admissions and hospital deaths. The future stretched out with no end in sight.

The light bulb turned on. I could keep working sixteen-hour days and every third night for the rest of my career, but things wouldn't change unless we figured how to motivate people to boil their water, immunize their children, build latrines, space their children, and adopt twenty or so other important health practices.

So we started a community health program. In our visits to other community programs in Kenya, it became apparent that most programs had a great understanding of the principles with good staff and significant funding. Yet, most of them were not seeing significant change. They didn't know how to motivate people. We returned to Tenwek and began to think, "What could we do differently to make it work better?" (We'll spend more time talking about the details of this community health program in a later chapter.)

God doesn't waste anything He brings into our lives. During college, I spent two summers working for the Bible company Southwestern, selling Bibles and other books door-to-door in Illinois and Pennsylvania. Along with hundreds of other college students, I worked twelve to thirteen hours a day strictly on commission. Doors were slammed in my face, dogs chased me, and Mormon customers tried to convert me when I visited their homes. Today, one of my most prized possessions is my "Gold Award" certificate from that summer. It is on my wall next to my diplomas stating that I worked 75 or more hours a week.

When I considered how to motivate people in Africa, I thought back to how Southwestern motivated their employees those two summers. I began to read books on what made the best companies in the U.S. successful. I condensed what I learned into five principles we applied to our community health program—and ultimately to our entire hospital system.

Let me lay the groundwork for what I'm about to share. Everyone has the same basic desires. Before focusing on anything else, a person wants to make sure they have food, clothing, shelter, and safety. Lacking any one of these, they will turn their attention to fulfilling that basic need. Basic needs are highly motivational, but what do you do when the issue goes beyond that?

What about money? Actually, it doesn't motivate people. No one thinks they are ever paid enough no matter how much their salary is raised. Money is in fact a de-motivator if it doesn't meet people's basic needs or is not given equitably. People work hard or change their behavior based on more intangible issues.

What is the common framework found in successful organizations?

People at all levels need to believe that:
1. What they do is important and makes a difference.
2. They are or can be the best at what they do.
3. The organization must ruthlessly protect and promote its key values.
4. The organization must be action-oriented. Small actions moving towards a goal are better than grandiose, time-consuming planning.
5. Everyone in the organization must be highly motivated.

Providing healthcare is obviously important and makes a big difference in people's lives. That is an easy concept to "sell" to our staff. We have a huge advantage over Coca-Cola executives. They have to convince their employees and their customers that Coke is life transforming. Of course, with millions of advertising dollars, they do just that. If you want to be happy, beautiful, or successful, just drink Coke!

I remember "preaching" to my staff that we were going to be the best mission hospital in Africa. My record was stuck in that groove. If I said it once, I said it a thousand times until the staff believed it and made it a reality.

Motivating people is the hardest thing of all to do. Here are the five most basic motivation principles I use with some examples and techniques from our community health work. Applications may vary because of culture, education, and other factors, but the principles remain the same no matter what you do or where you serve.

Foster a Sense of Healthy Pride
Identity - People have an innate desire to be recognized. That is why we have uniforms for Boy Scouts, the military, doctors, and nurses. Whether it is scrubs or a white coat, doctors and nurses have a specific look that sets them apart. Identity doesn't have to be a certain form of dress. In fact, uniforms in Kenya were associated with government employees and people were afraid of them. So we obtained a bright florescent red flight bag and put our logo on it for community health helpers (CHHs) to carry their teaching materials. They glowed so you could recognize them clear across the valley. We also designed and made large buttons for CHHs to wear that let people know who they were. We had a meaningful logo and publicized what it meant

throughout the community. We created a "brand" that meant something so our health helpers were known and admired because they wore it.

Respect - We took every opportunity to praise and recognize our team members. We always had the most important person we could find hand out training certificates at graduation ceremonies. Recognition by significant others is important. We invited and sometimes paid for transportation so family and friends could attend graduation exercises.

Sense of Worthiness - I was always trying to catch people doing something good. When I did, I wrote a letter on nice stationary to the district officer or chief lauding the person who had succeeded and copied the letter to the volunteer. I also continually told them how important and significant their work was to the program.

Facilitate Excellent Communication
Formal – Frequent communication at all levels is a great motivator. People want to know what is going on and how they fit in to the grand scheme. So we started printing a monthly newspaper distributed to every health helper and committee member. Each community also had monthly meetings of their committee and health helpers so they could communicate about what was happening. Each supervisor was responsible for communicating personally with each health helper and committee member that they worked with every month.

Informal – We encouraged cross-pollination between committees and health workers. Each month, I asked supervisors to give me the name of a committee member or health helper who needed encouragement or recognition. I wrote them a personal note on a post card with a great picture they would want to put on the wall.

Enable Non-Threatening Comparison
People want to know if they "fit in" and where they stand in relation to others. In medical school, they used to report our test scores by student number on a sheet posted on the bulletin board after exams. The first thing I did was to see what my score was. And the second thing was what? Of course, I looked at the other scores to see where my score fit in with the rest of the class.

Each month in our newspaper we published tables noting every CHH's activities in seven key areas. How many home visits and revisits did they make the previous month? How many new latrines were dug? You get the idea. We didn't have to say anything about performance because it was obvious who was working and who was not. Plus, everyone else knew how well everyone else was doing. Peer pressure can be a wonderful thing!

We summarized our data for each community so a committee could compare the results with other groups. We quickly learned that "what gets measured gets done." All I had to do was change a reporting category in the newspaper and volunteers would work much harder to improve in that area.

Facilitate Competition
That everyone can win – These contests measure effort and reward meeting minimum standards.

To recognize the highest performance – If you achieved the most new family planning users or had the highest number of latrines built, you received a certificate or a special button to wear. We also recognized a CHH of the month and a committee of the month.

Competition increases performance but also allows recognition. It is not what you give but how you give it that counts. If I handed you a pen because you are the best doctor or nurse, you might say thanks and put it in your pocket. If I gave it to you at the CMDA National Convention in front of all your colleagues, it would be more meaningful. If I took you to the White House and had the president give you the pen on national TV stating that you "have written a new chapter in international healthcare," you would frame it and keep it forever. The pen is worth the same, but the way it was given and its symbolism give it greater or lesser value.

This is the way we motivated the community members to change their health. We created a "Healthy Home Certificate" with lots of color, a red ribbon, and a gold seal. It looked like someone had graduated from the main university! If a home inspection confirmed a family changed five key health behaviors, we had the chief call the entire family up before the village to hand out one of the certificates I had signed. It cost only pennies to create and print. Families put their certificate on the wall, proudly showing it to their neighbors. The first year we gave out a few hundred, but soon the numbers increased to thousands each year. We created a second level certificate to encourage families to change five more behaviors. This simple idea did more to improve health than almost anything else we did.

We employed the same principles with our trained supervisors who were paid employees. We were having trouble getting reports in on time. We asked what they really wanted to do that they had never done before. They said they would love to fly in an airplane. We arranged a competition where everyone could win a ride in the small plane that brought visiting doctors to the hospital. We gave them money for busfare to travel back from Nairobi to the hospital. The supervisors who won talked about the experience for months.

Create A Sense of Family

Belonging – We had a great slogan, "Bir Mat Ko Lo," which meant "prevent the fire while it is still far." It was so popular that CHHs used it instead of the regular greeting when they shook hands with other community health people. We shouted it together at group meetings. It was almost the "secret club handshake" because it said you belonged to the family.

We are going to do this together – Everyone's ideas and critiques were sought and valued. This wasn't the hospital's program; this was our "family's" outreach.

We fostered:
- Shared experiences – We had huge celebrations/parties once or twice a year where everyone came together for education, recognition, and celebration.
- Shared rituals – Our greetings and many other things we did together became highly valued.
- Shared privileges – If you were part of the community health family, my door was open to you at any time, you got to go to the front of the clinic line at the hospital, etc.
- Shared responsibility – As health helpers and committees matured, they were increasingly emancipated just as you do as your kids grow up.

- Shared recognition – We gave the community and the volunteers all the credit.

You can employ these same principles with your colleagues, your staff, and your patients. Motivating people is one of the hardest but most necessary components of leadership. If you want to influence and change people, it's a skill you need to develop.

CHAPTER 3
COMMUNICATION ESSENTIALS

Without good communication skills, it is impossible to be a good leader. The problem is amplified when you work cross-culturally in your healthcare outreach. Words and gestures have different meanings or nuances that make good communication a long-term learning process! In our tribal group, pointing with your finger was considered rude so you pointed with your lips. I still get a laugh in the U.S. when someone catches me doing it when my hands are full!

Have you ever turned the wrong way down a one-way street? Bedlam results. The same is true if you treat a two-way street as a one-way thoroughfare. Unfortunately, many communicators do not realize that communication is a two-way street. It involves both the sender of the message and a recipient.

If you have kids or a spouse, you should know this already! Have you ever had to repeat yourself over and over again for your kids to listen? If I am sitting in the den reading a paper or a good book, I often tune out everything else around me. My wife Jody could call me for supper and I won't even hear her. Or I would say, "In a minute, honey." Then I get lost in what I am reading and five minutes later she calls me again. Sometimes the targets of the communication are not listening, do not correctly hear, or misinterpret what is said.

The good news is that you can learn to be a good communicator if you follow a few basic principles and practice them. If you do, you will avoid many of the problems that follow poor communication—misunderstandings, distrust, failure to accomplish important tasks or goals, and much more.

Principle 1 - Evoke not just a generic response, but a specific communication back to you that lets you know the recipient heard the message, understood and accepts it, and, if appropriate, will act upon it in a timely manner.

How do you do that in a hospital, clinic, or community health setting? Provide a method and expect a response to your communication if it is an important one. Let's say the hospital is struggling financially and you have to let staff go. You could make an announcement over the public address system, write a memo, or call a meeting with all the staff to break the news. Which option allows timely feedback? Obviously a meeting is the best option because it gives an opportunity for feedback from the participants. There can be clarifying questions. You can get a feel of how they are accepting the message and adjust your communication as needed.

Principle 2 - Use the appropriate communication method that best facilitates accomplishing your communication goal.

I send numerous e-mails each day because it offers the quickest turn around and is cheap. (Thank God my mom insisted I take typing in high school!) But e-mail is a lousy form of communication for dealing with major issues, sensitive discussions, or conflict. I was talking to some missionaries the other day, and their mission had decided to sell their headquarters and was considering merging with another organization. It was startling information which could significantly affect each individual, yet it was communicated via an e-mail to missionaries around the world. If you received that information, wouldn't you have questions? These missionaries did, but they were not able to ask them. The mission picked the wrong method to communicate important information.

E-mail and other forms of written communication do not show body language, express tone of voice, or allow immediate feedback. The more critical or concerning the communication, the more personalized it needs to be. If nothing else in this situation, the mission should have made the announcement to a large gathering of staff and missionaries and followed up with an audio or even video attachment to an e-mail sent to distant staff. This puts a person's expressions, tone of concern, and presence into a sensitive communication. That person should offer to answer questions and clarify the communication. Bottom line, tailor the communication vehicle to the weight of the communication being given. If you are putting out the call schedule for next month, it can be written. If you are assigning one doctor to take twice as much call as anyone else, you better talk to that doctor in person.

Fight the tendency most people have to avoid conflict by impersonally delivering bad or disturbing news. Even good leaders will avoid this snake, but be aware that it always comes back to bite you.

Oh, did I mention that the communication from the mission organization was not even sent by the mission president? To make matters worse, he gave that assignment to someone else and left the country on a previously scheduled trip, so he was not even available to answer questions.

Principle 3 - The appropriate person should deliver the communication.

If you are a physician, you never instruct the nurse to tell the patient, "The doctor told me to tell you that you have incurable cancer and will likely die in six months." The doctor has to convey that significant information face to face with appropriate time for discussion and questions.

Using the appropriate person works in the reverse as well. Do not diminish the authority of the person giving the communication by stepping in inappropriately. Recently I became aware that staff members in one of my departments were seen leaving work at all times during the day and sometimes leaving early from work. I could have called a meeting with that department and read the staff the riot act. Instead, I called in the department director to find out what was going on. Sometimes the staff members were going out on legitimate errands that prevented them from keeping to their work hours. I asked the director to deal with it, thereby strengthening his authority and giving him an opportunity to monitor the ongoing situation. I held him accountable and he held his staff to the rules. To leave a document trail, he wrote each staff member a note and then met with them as a group to further reinforce his communication and to listen to and answer their questions. Behavior changed, the appearance of wrong-doing was ameliorated by letting the receptionist know where they were going, and everyone was happier.

Principle 4 - Work hard to be empathetic with your listeners.

Where are the people you are trying to communicate with on this issue? How can you bridge from where they are to where you want to take them? For example, let's say you are having a major problem with keeping your facility clean. Kids are playing in and ruining the bushes, the latrines are a mess, trash is strewn around, and that's not the worst of it. Memos telling the staff to keep the hospital clean have not worked. No one likes cleaning up other people's trash or feces.

True, but how can you get your staff to take ownership of the problem? You call a meeting and start from a different place. You say, "Last week my wife and I had a wonderful dinner over at nurse Koech's home. She cooked a wonderful meal and her house and garden were so neat and orderly. We were impressed and I bet each one of you would have prepared food and cleaned up just like she did if you had invited us over to your home. In the same way, when we are working in the hospital, it is our house. We live and eat in the hospital for a good part of the day. I suspect like me, you have been embarrassed when officials or friends come by and see how messy and dirty 'our house' is. It is hard to keep our house clean when we have so many patients, but working together we can have a clean hospital that we all can be proud of. Here is the plan I have laid out to do just that. Let's discuss and improve on it and then…"

Get the idea? Your communication is more likely to be received and acted upon if you start from where the listeners are or from what they already know and believe. That is why you talk differently to children than adults. It is why you use simpler words with someone uneducated than with a colleague. Your communication should start from where the listeners are in their knowledge, experience, and beliefs.

Principle 5 - More is communicated non-verbally than verbally.

Tone, volume, pacing, and gestures communicate much more than the actual words. I can say, "I love you" with a tone of endearment, a question mark, or even an angry tone as I push myself away from my spouse.

I came back after furlough to a crisis at Tenwek. The staff was demanding the dismissal of the matron, pay increases, and much more. The board met, addressed the issues, and communicated its decision to the staff. The doctor in charge left, leaving me in charge. Three days later, a hospital employee came to tell me the staff wanted to meet with me, pulling me away from dinner guests at 7:30 in the evening. When I arrived, the hospital meeting room was packed, every seat was full, and several staff members were standing. On a slip of paper, I was presented with the same list of demands the board had already dealt with. I read the first couple of demands and the threat to strike, folded the paper, and put it in my pocket. I put my hands in my pockets to look relaxed (which I was not) and then in a calm but firm voice said, "If Tenwek Hospital is such a bad place to work, I encourage you to quit and go find another job." I then calmly walked out and went back to finish dinner. My words called their bluff, and my attitude and gestures showed I was not concerned by the threats. As far as I was concerned, the matter was finished.

The next day everyone was at work and the issues were never brought up again. (Whew!) In retrospect, I believe my non-verbal communication was more powerful than my words. Walking out sent a clear message that there was not going to be any negotiating on decisions already made by the board.

Principle 6 - Develop the skill of listening and interpreting.

Most of my communication mistakes were made because I did not listen well or take time to collect all the facts. Others occurred because I spoke when I was angry or upset. After my second term when I had been in charge of Tenwek, built a hydro plant, started a nursing school and a community development program, and generally burnt myself out, I got a letter from my field director. It said, "Dave, I was doing the yearly assessments on the missionaries at Tenwek, and a good number of people felt like you were much more interested in getting things done than in the welfare of the people involved."

Whoa, was I angry! "He hadn't taken call every third or fourth night, seen one hundred patients a day and managed a staff of four hundred," I mentally ranted. "No other missionary came close to accomplishing what I did the last four years, and this is my thanks?" By the grace of God, I did not write him back right away. The letter would have probably auto-combusted! After venting to my wife, reflection, and prayer, God broke through my pride and emotional barriers. I admitted he was right. I had focused too much on the problems and not enough on the people. As we later communicated, I learned my lesson and changed my management style, hopefully for a lifetime.

It is impossible to take back things wrongly said. Learn to listen well, collect the facts from all those involved, and make an effort to learn to read non-verbal communication cues. As you master these disciplines, you will do a much better job of interpreting what is going on and communicating the right thing.

Principle 7 - Use examples, stories, slogans, and analogies to get your point across.

Once a year, we hold media training where I teach doctors how to do media interviews. One of the most important things they learn is the power of a sound bite, example, story, or analogy. They are powerful communication tools, especially in many of the cultures where missionaries work. That is how the local people learn and understand.

One of the ways to motivate people is through competitions, and we had lots of them in our community health program. Using these non-financial incentives turbocharged the work efforts of our volunteers. Some competitions only had one winner. Others allowed everyone to win if they met a minimum set of standards. One year, the prizes were bags of special seed corn, and we gave out the prizes at our big community health event. In front of the hundreds of people at the event, I told a story and drew the analogy between the work of planting, tilling, and harvesting and what they were doing in their efforts to plant seeds of health in the community. Everyone went home with their prizes; more importantly, they went away telling everyone that they were "health seed planters" as they showed off their prizes.

Get the idea? You want to drive home the message, make it personal, and make it memorable. Testimony, stories, slogans, and analogies punch your message through mental barriers and get your point across to your audience.

Principle 8 - Maintain a positive attitude.

Your attitude carries weight. You want to lead, not drive people through your communication if at all possible. Pick your words and tones carefully to convey a positive attitude, even in a negative situation. Let's say you have to lay people off. The number of patients has declined, so income is not meeting projections. Instead of saying you are downsizing, you may want to use "right-sizing," a corporate term which is more positive. Communicate the benefits this move will bring for the future of the hospital, but more importantly for the remaining staff. "Once we right-size, we will be able to improve the benefits for our remaining staff members. It is difficult to let some of you go, but I am going to do all we can to ease the transition. God will see us through this time. He is still in control."

Even negative news can be conveyed in positive terms. When it is over, you want staff to think, "This was difficult for him. He cares about us and better days are ahead."

Principle 9 - Be consistent.

Dr. Ernie Steury served as the Executive Director and I was the Medical Superintendent for a number of years when we were at Tenwek together. Like children do with parents, staff who didn't like my answer would go to Ernie to try and get a different one, and vice versa. We learned that we needed to be in constant communication to make sure people did not divide and conquer us. We worked hard to speak with one voice, to be consistent. The same is true even if the communication only comes from you. You will get in trouble if you tell one group one thing and another group something different, or if you change your position without acknowledging or explaining the change.

The other reason for being consistent is that studies show it can take up to seven different communications to get someone to change a habit. Stay on message and repeat it as necessary. It is one of the keys to good communication.

Principle 10 - Develop trust.

No matter how well you communicate, you have to have trust. The listener has to give you the benefit of the doubt. If you communicate with someone who does not trust you (and you know what I mean), that person filters everything through a series of misconceptions and puts everything you communicate in the worst light.

Remember the story about the hospital staff ready to go on strike? I unwittingly started the fracas when I wrote an orientation manual for visiting staff. In that manual, I advised visitors to not give gifts to national staff members without first checking with a missionary. They did not realize an old pair of jeans was worth a month's salary or that some staff had the goal of getting close with visitors so they could milk each one for gifts. This was causing jealousy and hard feelings.

One of our visitors left the orientation manual in the surgery dressing room and an OR assistant with a chip on his shoulder took it. His interpretation of this section was that the missionaries wanted to oppress the nationals. He stirred up problems all over the hospital with his "evidence" in hand. As a result, trust broke down and near anarchy followed.

Lack of trust is one of the main reasons interpersonal conflicts start and persist. Trust takes a long time to earn, but only seconds to lose. Consistency, sincerity, and actions matching your words will build trust over time. With hard cases, one on one communication, confrontation, and discipline may be necessary.

Remember, what you put in writing can come back to haunt you. It is "hard evidence," so be very careful when you put things in writing. If it is a sensitive communication, have one or two other people read it and give you feedback. What you think you are saying may not be how others interpret it.

Communication is an art. Some people are innately great communicators, but most of us have to learn to do it well. Take these principles and apply them. Realize that every communication is a learning experience on how to do it better. With effort, practice, and attention to detail, you can become a better communicator.

CHAPTER 4
PRESENTING A HEART-CHANGING MESSAGE

Some people are naturally gifted speakers, but most are not. Even if you include yourself in the latter category, you can still learn to communicate effectively. As a missionary, it is worth the effort because you need to communicate well with those you lead and you will need to speak frequently when you are on home assignment. If you are already serving, you learned this the hard way!

Like becoming a great golfer, the best way to learn to speak well is to practice, but first you need to learn the fundamentals. Let's start by answering a few questions to help you present a heart-changing message on home assignment.

What is your purpose?
You want to accomplish five things when speaking about missions. Let's start with the least important. First, you want to inform the audience by telling them what you are doing or will do. Unfortunately, many missionaries get stuck here, creating a boring travelogue or laundry list of daily activities. Though you must inform, it is more important to make it interesting for your listeners.

Secondly, if you are returning and speaking to supporters of your ministry, you want to report how their prayers and financial support are making a difference. The key is not just to report activities but to tell how their investments have saved souls and changed lives. You want to let them know they have changed lives for now and for eternity.

You also have the purpose of building relationships. You want the audience to feel like they know you and you want them to like you. One of your primary jobs on home assignments is to build friendships. You want individuals to identify with you and stand in your shoes for a while, as if they were walking with you as a missionary.

I remember my first deputation message. The first third of the message focused on sharing our spiritual journey to serving overseas to allow the audience to get to know our family. I knew people were asking in their minds, "Why would you decide to do this?" It was a great opportunity for our listeners to learn about our family background, call, preparation, struggles, and mission experience.

When it came to telling about the ministry, I tried to have the audience walk in my shoes. I asked them to imagine that we just landed a 747 in the church parking lot so all of us could get on board and travel to Tenwek. I would then have them walk through the gates of the hospital with me, take them on rounds on the ward and introduce them to typical or memorable patients. I wanted it to feel like they had journeyed to Kenya and we had experienced something together. So thirdly, shared experiences build relationships. I wanted each individual in the congregation to live our lives and ministry with us so they would want us to be their missionaries.

The fourth purpose is even more important. You want to inspire your listeners. You want to create a passion in them to reach the world for Christ. To do that, they need to understand the need and be moved to do something about it. You want them to internalize the challenges you face and see them as projects they need to do something about through prayer, financial support, or coming alongside and working with you. Quotations or slogans from others can be helpful in accomplishing this.

- "If Jesus Christ be God and died for me, then no sacrifice can be too great for me to make for Him." - C.T. Studd
- "God's work done in God's way will never lack God's supplies." - J. Hudson Taylor
- "I have found that there are three stages in every great work of God; first, it is impossible, then it is difficult, then it is done." - J. Hudson Taylor

The fifth purpose is to challenge them. By challenge them, I mean bring them to an action point of actually doing something about the issues you raised. Sympathy without action doesn't change a thing. The challenge is often at the end of your message as you use a story or illustration to challenge them to get involved.

Who is your audience?
Once you understand your purpose, you need to ask this question. One message doesn't fit all. Your content, length, points, and challenge will be different for children, teenagers, adults, or senior citizens. Your message will change if you talk to a medical audience versus a non-medical audience. Your illustrations will be different if you speak to an elderly Sunday school class than to a youth group. Tailoring your message to the right audience is key. When possible, ask for more information about the audience from your contact person. If you are speaking to the entire church body at a main service, check out the church's website to learn more about it. I remember speaking in a church where I was the first missionary to stand in the pulpit in more than thirty years. At another church, I was just one of many multiple missionary speakers in the past twenty years. Tailor your message to your audience so you can take them from where they are to where they need to be.

Your next job is to plan your message. This could be writing it word for word, but most people sound more personal and unscripted with an outline as opposed to a manuscript. I start with an introduction using a quip, joke, or humorous story to build rapport with the audience. Make sure the humor is appropriate and transitions well into your message. Depending on how I begin the main body of the message, I will then pause for prayer to set the tone for the message.

Grab the audience's attention early. The best way is with a gripping story, quandary, or question. My first missionary message started out with the question, "What does it mean to deny yourself? Is it saying, 'No!' to a second piece of pie? Or did Christ mean something else when He said, 'Deny yourself, take up your cross and follow me?'" I then added, "I remember the first time He asked me if I was willing to deny myself," and then launched into my testimony.

It is also important to theme your message. You probably still remember Tony Compolo's famous message, "It is Friday but Sunday's Coming." Why? Because it had a memorable theme. I remember hearing a great missionary message a few years ago with the provoking theme, "The Doctor Must Die." It still sticks in my mind because of its theme.

Your theme and/or major points should have scriptural support. Your message can be built around one Scripture or you can have a number sprinkled throughout your key points. Most messages can be built around one to five key supporting points to establish your theme. I use a military analogy when I preach a message with the theme, "God's Special Forces." In this message, I talk about the five characteristics necessary to "go behind enemy lines" to carry the gospel—commitment, loyalty, training, compassion, and boldness.

It is illustrative to understand how Christ so effectively spoke His message. He stated a principle and then shared a story (parable) to drive the point home. People learn best through stories. That is why a good illustration is worth its weight in gold. When sharing a story, carry the people there by painting a picture with words. There is a difference in impact between saying, "I was trying to send a message on our satellite fax machine" and saying, "It was a sultry night with gunshots and grenade explosions punctuating the night sky of Mogadishu as I crouched to escape observation below the low parapet of our roof to send an important message on our satellite fax machine."

Hear the difference? One sentence transports you to the situation and the other does not.

Another way to make your point is with an analogy—a comparison between two things similar in some respects which is used to help explain the topic and make it easier to understand. I use an analogy explaining how God can make and mold us by describing how unattractive crude oil is, but once it is purified and molded it can make artificial lenses to replace those removed in cataract operations. Like the oil, we have to be purified under pressure and molded into something useful by Christ.

You will also probably want to share some numbers, but compare and contrast those numbers to make them meaningful. When I talked about Tenwek's catchment area, I didn't just say we served 300,000 people. I would find out the population of a city nearby to where I spoke and compare it. If I were speaking in Bristol, Tennessee, I would say, "Imagine a population eight times the size of Bristol with only three doctors to meet the needs." Another option is to contrast a number with a U.S. norm. "There is one doctor for every 500 people in the U.S. Where I serve, there is one for every 100,000." Percentages are dry and sterile, so don't use them. Instead of saying 10 percent of the people in your country have AIDS, say something like this, "If you walk down the street in our capital city, one out of every ten people you pass is carrying the deadly AIDS virus."

Visual aids punch your message home. I still remember a chaplain from a federal penitentiary who spoke at my high school. He was telling a dramatic story of a prisoner being stabbed with a homemade knife, called a "shive." When he got to the climax of the story, he pulled the actual "shive" out of his pocket and stabbed it into the top of the podium. I can still see it quivering forty years later! One of our teachers spoke on "using your ajoinings of time," and flicked quarters into the audience as she talked about wasting time being like wasting money. I know a missionary doctor who dresses up like a Masaii and delivers his message from the Masaii's perspective. All of these are visual methods to reinforce your theme and get your message across.

Slides can be used as visual aids, but they need to be of good quality and you need to keep them moving. When I showed slides, I used two projectors and showed a total of 140 slides in ten minutes. Of course in this day and time, a video is often most appropriate. A video needs to be well produced, short, and memorable.

After you plan your message, practice it. The more you give the message, the better you will do. As you practice, keep it moving. Don't get bogged down with a story that is too detailed. Time yourself and work on giving your message in different lengths. If it is a thirty-minute message, what are you going to cut out if the pastor tells you three minutes before the service begins that you only have twenty minutes to speak?

Get critiques of your message from knowledgeable people—pastors, other missionaries, etc.—on how you can make your message better. I encourage people to go through the painful process of listening to themselves or watching a visual recording of their presentations. If you do this, get someone to sit down and watch it with you to give feedback.

Here are a few practical pointers.

- After you complete your outline, highlight key words to stimulate your memory of the point. That way you can quickly look at your notes as you speak and keep track of where you are. I use different colors for main points, illustrations, and Scripture.
- Inject as much humor as you can into your presentation where appropriate. The best humor makes fun of yourself or helps other people make fun of themselves.
- To generate emotion, you need to feel the emotion you are wanting to generate. If you want them to be moved, you should be moved. If you want your audience to be passionate, you need to be.
- After the preparation, it is time to present your talk. Before you speak, bathe your presentation in prayer and get others to pray as well. God is the ultimate One to move hearts. You're not putting on a performance but letting Him use your voice and the Holy Spirit to speak through you. I always ask God to empty me of myself and fill me with His spirit before I speak.
- Keep within your time limits. Nothing will blow your credibility and distract from your message more than taking too much time.
- Don't just preach a message on the theology of missions. I've seen missionaries do that and the response is, "Our pastor could have done that and done a better job at it." People want to hear your stories and experiences. On the other hand, don't just tell stories and experiences without making a point.
- Move and use body language. Standing behind a pulpit can be boring. Use a wireless mike, move around the platform, and dramatize the stories you tell. When I tell the story of taking care of a woman and her child in a hovel in Mogadishu, I get down on my knee as I did when I was looking in the hovel. I act out the story as I tell it. Dramatizing your stories makes them much more effective and interesting.
- Reiterate your main points to drive them home. As someone said, "Tell them what you are going to say, say it, and then

tell them what you said." Repetition helps people remember. When I finish preaching, I want people to go away remembering just one to three things. Those are the things I want to punch home again and again.
- Make eye contact. The smaller the group, the more important the eye to eye contact with individuals. This is something you have to practice since looking people in the eye can be distracting to your thinking. It is worth the effort because it helps you to really connect with your audience.

If you don't have enough good stories or illustrations, collect them from others or read missionary biographies. A year or so after preaching at a large church, I saw a missionary executive who had been at the meeting. He said, "I loved that message you gave. I've been preaching it all across the U.S.!" Imitation is the nicest form of flattery, but I had to ask, "Where?" I didn't want to visit one of the churches he had spoken at and preach the same message!

Public speaking is one of your greatest privileges and most important opportunities. There is nothing more gratifying than to see God using you to help transform someone's life. With purpose, planning, and practice, you can become a more effective speaker.

CHAPTER 5
IGNORE THE GRAPEVINE AND IT WILL HANG YOU

The hardest thing about missionary life is being so far away from family. Back before cell phones, computers, and Skype, I kept in contact with family through a shortwave radio. Yes, I was one of those people with a 60-foot homemade tower outside my concrete block house with a big tri-band antenna perched on top. When work allowed on Saturday afternoons, I would power up my Kenwood transceiver and talk to "hams" around the world. Hopefully one of them would be a friend in my home town who would call my parents over to his "radio shack." I got to touch home and they got to hear the delightful things their grandchildren were doing! This innocent hobby brought "home" closer.

I say innocent because some nationals in our area didn't perceive it as such. They spread rumors through the local "grapevine," that path of communication where news, gossip, or rumors pass unofficially from person to person. And the implausibility of the rumors grew with each transmission—"Dr. Stevens is communicating with the CIA," became "the missionaries have guns hidden underwater in the river," to finally "they are planning to overthrow the government." Rumors became "facts" until Criminal Investigation Department officers showed up, searched my home, and confiscated all my radio equipment despite the framed Kenya radio license hanging on my wall. I did not complain too much; I was just glad they had not put me in prison!

The problem wasn't the local grapevine. The problem was I had ignored it. If you ignore the local grapevine, it will hang you. I've seen it in missionary institutions, community programs, and even among missionary colleagues. In fact, the longer you ignore the grapevine, the quicker it will get its revenge on you.

You ignore the grapevine by:

- Not acknowledging it exists.
- Not realizing its power.
- Not being attached to the vine.
- Not feeding it.

People love to talk and speculate. Not only do they speculate, but they assume. Your good friends always assume you have the best motives and intentions. Those who don't like you always assume you are up to something bad. Though the majority of people fall in the middle of that spectrum, they are not the silent majority. They all pass the message down the line and are strongly influenced by what they hear through unofficial channels. The grapevine is always on and functioning because everyone has a desire to be on the "inside" and know what is going on.

Knowledge is power. Those who don't like you or are just suspicious by nature regularly feed the grapevine with their own assertions and sometimes outright lies. The more sensational the information, the greater their alleged power, and the faster the story travels. Those in the middle are negatively influenced and don't usually share what they heard with your friends, so it doesn't get back to you until you have a huge problem. You may only recognize a few rumblings before the eruption that can badly damage you or your ministry.

The closer people are in proximity, the faster the transmission speed. Institutions where staff members congregate daily are notorious for active grapevines that don't stop when staff members leave the premises. Staff members carry what they heard home to their families, their communities, and sometimes to the authorities.

A nurse at our hospital was loved by our staff and she loved to joke with them and vice versa. One day at the end of some banter, she said in a joking way, "See you later alligator, after while crocodile." A staff member who was present immediately connected to the grapevine and spread the word that the nurse was calling national staff animals, a deep insult in the Kipsigis culture. The sensational accusation reached all the way to authorities in Nairobi, six hours by car. Within days, threats of deportation followed until the waters were calmed.

I doubt I have to convince you about the grapevine. You probably have your own stories. You have experienced its power, a power further amplified by working cross-culturally. You cannot eliminate the grapevine, but you can get attached to it, learn to counter its negative effects, and even utilize it for your purposes. In today's vernacular, you can go "viral."

Here are the keys:

- Communicate, communicate, communicate.
- Locate a few good grapevine nodes.
- Preempt.
- Proactively keep the information flowing.

The best way to head off rumor, gossip, and innuendo is to constantly communicate formally through staff meetings, written information, and recruiting other authority figures to communicate your message. That means you must keep your leaders well informed and encourage them to speak out. You may want to create a communication "tree." Recently, we cancelled church due to snow. The person making that decision accessed the church phone tree and, within an hour or so, members were informed.

Part of communicating about controversial, easily misinterpreted, or crisis situations is deciding what messages you want to send down the grapevine. I remember watching a news report about a group of people watching a surfing event who were swept off some rocks while observing the competitors. The person in charge of the event had her message ready with four key points: "We had medical personnel there quickly; we told people to watch the webcast instead of coming when there were few safe places to observe the competition; we had a sign posted warning people not to stand on these rocks; and our hearts go out to those injured." She had a prepared and specific message that she delivered on national news, thereby effectively disarming her critics before they had time to poison the grapevine.

Ask yourself, what do people need to know? What questions or concerns would I have about this situation if I received this news? How can this information be twisted and what do I need to say to prevent that? How can I explain this in the most understandable way? You are only going to get one opportunity to give information the first time. Make sure you think it through and do it right.

Use the informal as well as formal communication network. Who are the effective nodes on the grapevine? What "inside" scoop can you give them that you want to be heard by everyone? Often the grapevine is more trusted than the formal communication network so don't neglect to feed it.

Here are a couple of caveats. If you have bad news, get all of it out there at once in the most comprehensive way possible. A few years ago, we had to lay off 20 percent of our staff for financial reasons. After making the termination decisions, I kept that information private. I met with all our staff to explain our financial situation, its implications, what we were planning to do, and that those affected would be notified in the next few hours so as not to drag out the pain. I explained the severance package and that we would work hard to help those affected find other jobs. I told them how I made the decision on who to let go. I emphasized they were selected not because they were doing a bad job, but because we had some redundancy in their areas of responsibility. I expressed my sorrow for those affected and optimism for the future—CMDA was going to do well after this "right-sizing" and those still employed were not in danger of losing their jobs. Then Dr. Rudd or I met personally with each person affected.

Get the idea? It was bad news, but I made sure I gave all the bad news at once, and answered questions before they were asked or before employees were tempted to feed the grapevine with speculations.

You also need to preempt or correct bad information traveling on the grapevine whenever possible. Remember the old Abbot and Costello comical sketch, "Who's on first?" When it comes to communication, you want to be.

That means you need to have your ears to the ground listening to what is on the grapevine. When you sense a problem, you want to get your communication engine revved up and send your message out. The longer you delay, the more damage the wrong information will have.

Years ago, a single national nurse in Kenya took an overdose of chloroquine in a failed abortion attempt. She killed her baby and herself. It was a tragedy that could have been made much worse by sensational stories on the grapevine. We called a staff meeting as quickly as possible to explain what happened and our efforts to save her life. We expressed God's love for her and her grieving relatives, and talked about how this type of tragedy could be prevented in the future. We flooded the grapevine with the facts and our concern so it was our message and not rumors that circulated around the hospital and in the community.

The best way to avoid being blindsided by the grapevine is to systemize and prioritize your formal and informal communication, both horizontally and vertically with your staff members. Don't ignore it!

PART 2
ETHICS

CHAPTER 6
MEDICAL MISSION BIOETHICS

It was funny and sad at the same time. I was preparing to speak at the Global Missions Health Conference in Louisville, Kentucky, on "Ethical Issues in Missionary Medicine." So I did a web search to see what else had been written on the topic. The only thing that came up was an advertisement—for my upcoming appearance in Louisville!

Of course, there are libraries full of articles and books on the ethics of cloning, stem cells, and abortion. There are good articles on the ethical issues of justice in the macro-allocation of healthcare resources. Yet, micro-allocation issues related to delivering healthcare in developing countries are seldom addressed. When they are, they don't address the unique situation found in mission hospitals. Perhaps those of us who have served in the overseas trenches are the best "experts" available. At least we have experienced the problems first-hand and wrestle with our decisions.

Unfortunately, with the incredible demands of missionary medicine, not much time is available for reflection. What principles should guide us as we decide who gets the last tank of oxygen, whether we should attempt a difficult surgery we have never done before, or whether we should charge higher fees to our wealthier patients? With the enormous disparity in education between doctor and patients, what about the issue of paternalism and informed consent?

An even more basic question is do we have the time to address these issues at all? I believe we should make the time. The issues we face are not theoretical. You are unlikely to ever have the opportunity to do stem cell research, but you will deal with ethical issues in your workplace every day. With more government and other third party funding for major programs, missionary facilities are facing more outside scrutiny. Even more important than our testimony to non-believers is making sure we are pleasing God in everything we do. We want to make decisions that are biblical and honor Him.

Let's lay down some context. The mission healthcare facility or training program is a unique entity. Missionary healthcare workers are highly committed, having left home, family, financial security, and familiarity to serve the poor and needy. They are highly educated and deeply care about the people God called them to serve. They tend to be isolated, focused, and overworked. They routinely have to deal with advanced pathology, inadequate diagnostic equipment, and therapeutic armamentarium. They provide healthcare that is better than most offered in the areas where they serve. They are not paid directly by their patients. They are rich in resources compared to those they treat. They often carry heavy administrative loads and are most likely in charge of their department or facility.

With that context, where do we begin to examine this large topic? A framework is helpful. In ethical circles, we refer to this as the "Georgetown Mantra." Four ethical principles exist which are really the secularization of the biblical principles that have existed for thousands of years.

1. Beneficence – Do good.
2. Non-malfeasance – Do no harm.
3. Autonomy – Let patients make their own informed decisions.
4. Justice – Be fair to all.

Biblical-based ethics are richer and fuller than secular ethics. For example, we are commanded not to just do good but to have our good works flow out of a heart of love (Galatians 6:10). We are told, "Love does no harm to its neighbor" (Romans 13:10a, NIV 1984). Christian ethics does not maintain that man is simply autonomous, but that he has a personal responsibility for his actions before God. The Bible teaches not just justice but grace—giving people what they don't deserve—because that is what God did for us.

All the same, the Georgetown Mantra offers a good platform to dive into ethics in missionary medicine. There is no doubt that medical missionaries want to be beneficent. The ethical issues in this area arise because of competing goods. Both are good efforts, but should I put my time into curative or preventative work? It is good to pay my national staff adequate wages, but it is also good to offer free treatment to the poor. If I do one, I may have trouble doing the other. There are many examples available, with some involving the lesser of two evils instead of the better of two goods.

1. You desperately need the medicines and supplies held up by customs in port. Patients will die without them so you go to deal with the situation. There is no duty on medicines but the customs official wants a "small gift" for facilitating the process. Which is the lesser of the two evils? Is it worse to let patients die for lack of medicines or to bribe an official?
2. You are short staffed and your doctors and nurses are burning out. If you let a doctor or nurse go on vacation, the wards won't be covered and some patients are likely to die. Yet, you risk losing missionary staff members if you delay vacations.
3. You are not well staffed, but you just received a shipment of donated monitoring equipment, infusion pumps, and respirators. Your missionary surgeon colleague wants to set up an ICU to take care of difficult cases. A number of patients who could have survived actually died due to lack of intensive care. You have so few trained nurses in your hospital that you are afraid pouring your scarce personnel into a few patients will be at the expense of the many.

When there are two competing goods or two evils, you may have to make your decision based on the principle of utility. Utilitarian ethics has a place in medicine under the right conditions. Adapted from Dr. John Feinberg, a philosophy/ethics professor at Trinity International University, they are:

1. There must be no moral absolutes for or against an action. For example, a twelve-year-old girl comes in with rabies and she will most likely die. Utilitarian ethics alone would allow you to give her a lethal injection to put her out of her misery. However, this violates the absolute principle that we should not kill; therefore, it is unacceptable to base your decision on utility. Most would say the moral absolute against giving or ac-

cepting bribes in Exodus 23:8 would not allow you to bribe a customs official to get medicines into the country.
2. There is a conflict between two moral duties and both cannot be fulfilled. For example, two patients desperately need emergency surgery. One has a 10 percent chance of survival and the other has a 50 percent chance of survival. You can't operate on both at the same time, so you decide based on survival probability.
3. You must prioritize your duties. You have to pick one patient to operate on first.
4. There are limited resources. Long before "managed care" in the U.S., missionary doctors had to deal with the issue of unlimited needs and limited resources.
5. When you know your moral duty but are not sure how to fulfill it.

When these criteria are met, you can use a utilitarian approach. You send your nurse or doctor on vacation knowing that losing them long-term will cause much more harm than allowing them to leave on a two-week vacation. You don't open an ICU to save a few when many more will die for lack of good nursing care. You give the only tank of oxygen to the patient most likely to survive.

Non-malfeasance, doing no harm, raises even thornier issues in missionary medicine. When practicing in the U.S. or other developed countries, you can be sure not to work beyond your training or experience by referring patients you could not comfortably handle. In missionary medicine, there is usually no one to refer to as you have the most expertise and are often the last resort. Again and again, you practice beyond your training, experience, equipment, nursing support, facility capacity, supplies, and the time you have to give to an individual patient.

Early in my career at Tenwek, I was the only doctor working one day when a man who had been cut by a machete through the maxilla was brought in for treatment. I did my first tracheostomy and put on my first set of arch bars as I turned the pages of a surgical text propped up by the operating table. Halfway through the case, they brought in the man's nephew who had also been attacked. His right arm and left hand were severed and he had cuts in his skull and back. With one operating room, I directed the medical student in completing his amputations while I operated on the first patient. When I finished, I noted he had a blown pupil, diagnosed a subdural, and put in my first burr holes with the nurse turning the page of the surgical atlas. We had no neurosurgeon to call. By the grace of God, both patients survived, but I was the first to admit I was working beyond my family practice training and experience.

What principles should guide the inexperienced and overwhelmed missionary doctor in this area? Where do we draw the line in doing no harm?

First, you should always defer to someone with more knowledge and expertise if you have that option. I had a boy come in who had been shot with a barbed arrow that penetrated from his descending colon to his kidney. The head of the arrow was buried in the spine. I couldn't pull the arrow back through the wound without massive damage. I couldn't pull it through because of the way it was wedged into the spine and I didn't have anything to cut the arrowhead. But a missionary surgeon with twenty years of experience was due back from safari in three hours, so I packed the wound and waited until he returned. He sterilized the bolt cutters from his toolbox and cut the head off! (Now why didn't I think of that?)

Secondly, you have to look at the consequence of inaction. A visiting orthopedist once refused to operate on a patient who badly needed his expertise because he didn't have every instrument he normally used in the U.S. He didn't want to take the risk of harming the patient when conditions weren't perfect, but the consequence was the loss of a leg or a less experienced surgeon doing the case. He failed to examine the consequences of doing nothing until we had a personal discussion.

Thirdly, you have to evaluate the risk and benefits of each situation. I didn't tackle taking out a hematoma already protruding through a patient's abdominal wall. The surgery was extremely risky and the benefit of taking out the tumor was very small. We decided not to operate on newborns with spina bifida who were paraplegic because they invariably died when they went home. Parents did not have the capability to take care of them in the village. We didn't pour scarce resources into a case we could technically do but had little benefit. We would just be harming the patient and saddling family members with a large bill.

Fourthly, the principle of malfeasance mandates that you seek change. If you have a large number of vesical-vaginal fistulas in your service area, you need to seek extra training to meet that need. The principle of doing no harm requires you to get training onsite or on furlough to provide the best care possible for the unfortunate patients needing your help.

Children at Tenwek regularly died due to lack of oxygen when they had pneumonia and other respiratory diseases. It was difficult to transport oxygen tanks eighty kilometers over muddy roads and those tanks were expensive. We were obligated to seek change because children were harmed for lack of oxygen. We obtained an industrial oxygen concentrator plant since we couldn't afford a medical unit and modified it to provide a safe source of piped oxygen to our patients.

Autonomy is a more insidious issue in missionary medicine due to the disparity of education between medical staff and patients. The problem is compounded by language barriers. We "know" what is best for patients. Our desire to help, advise, and protect may cause us to neglect individual choice and the patient's personal responsibility to make decisions. The patient's worldview also causes difficulty. For someone with an animistic worldview, an anatomical explanation of appendicitis makes little sense. They are convinced they have been cursed by someone or their disease is the result of evil spirits. They want to be cut so you can release the spirit causing their pain. The time required to get informed consent also conspires against the missionary doctor. You simply don't have time to get informed consent for everything you do.

Yet the Bible says, "Do nothing out of selfish ambition or vain conceit, but in humility consider others better than yourselves" (Philippians 2:3, NIV 1984). As missionary doctors, we have the responsibility to get informed consent as best we can for general anesthetics, serious procedures, and expensive therapies. The level of consent required depends on the educational level of your patients and the location of your service area. A missionary doctor in a more developed country or urban area may have different requirements than someone working in the jungles of the Congo. Of course, you need to meet the standard of the country in which you practice.

Missionary doctors also run the risk of having too much autonomy themselves. Many work with no risk of malpractice and little or no accountability from their colleagues. That is why it is important to set up measuring systems to monitor activities and outcomes. What are the trends in your C-section or mortality rates from year to year? How do your statistics compare to other mission, government, or private hospitals in your country? I also recommend morbidity and mortality conferences and case reviews of bad outcomes. You should always be asking the question, how could we have done better? All of us need to be accountable spiritually and professionally to others.

It is also healthy to visit other facilities to learn from them or have a consultant come in to evaluate your patient care, management system, and programs. Too often, missionary hospitals and doctors operate in isolation with each trying to recreate the wheel. Much can be learned from comparison with other ministries and through cross-pollination.

It is also helpful to periodically get feedback from the community you serve through formal or informal surveys, patient questionnaires, or exit interviews. You need to know how the people you serve see your services.

The last issue in missionary medical ethics is justice. We need to be fair as we make our decisions with resources and our time allocations in patient care. We also need to pay our staff reasonable wages. One area where this crops up is, should a mission hospital provide "private" services and charge higher rates? This is often done to generate income for the self-supporting mission facility so they can provide reduced or free care for the truly needy. Is this a just system?

It can be if it does not affect the basic quality of care. Every patient deserves a timely diagnosis and treatment, but private patients can be charged more for shorter waiting times in a clinic, private rooms, or a more elaborate hospital diet. On the other hand, it would be unethical to allow a less urgent surgical patient to pay to "jump the queue" before a patient who needs emergency treatment. This is not only true for those who can pay but also for the powerful with political clout. This is often a delicate situation, but we must remember people are watching and we are commanded to be "respecters of persons." We must be as fair and impartial as the situation reasonably allows.

One of the ethical theory systems gaining credence in the U.S. is called virtue ethics. Its thrust is that the best way to ensure an ethical decision in medicine is to have it made by a virtuous person. I think this is especially true for Christians. Luke 10:27 states, "...'Love the Lord your God with all your heart and with all your soul and with all your strength and with all your mind'; and, 'Love your neighbor as yourself'" (NIV 1984). If you live your life by this verse, you will weigh every decision in the balance of the Great Physician's teaching.

Here are some practical recommendations.

- Form a group representative of your staff, church, and community to consider ethical issues if you are practicing in a larger facility.
- On important issues, write out principles, policies, and guidelines. It will help you and others make decisions. Start out with the more important issues. Obtain documents from other hospitals to guide you.
- Communicate your policies to all levels of staff and allow a mechanism for feedback.
- Put a system into place for reviewing specific cases. There is knowledge in wise counsel.
- Periodically review your policies and update them.

We admonish our staff at the end of every chapel as they return to work to, "Go and be godly!" Sound ethical advice for all of us who work to live out the Great Commission.

CHAPTER 7
SHORT-TERM ETHICS

I'm sure my title caught your attention. Rest easy. I'm not suggesting your ethics should be short-term! The title actually was prompted by a longer title in the *Journal of the American Medical Association* which was brought to my attention by a missionary friend. It is entitled "Ethical Considerations for Short-term Experiences by Trainees in Global Health."

The article is worth a read, but it is not a free download. It does raise some issues worth thinking about that I want to address. It notes that almost two out of every three U.S. medical schools have established global health initiatives with the goal of reducing disparities through research, education, and service. Often due to student demand, these medical schools are now providing rotations in "resource limited settings." The article lauds these as noble goals but raises ethical cautions about when schools go beyond classroom teaching to providing field experience.

My first medical mission experience occurred after my junior year in college. I had no clinical skills or knowledge, but a handful of staff in a bush hospital setting trained me to pass instruments in surgery and deliver a baby. Of course, the baby was from a grand multiparous woman so the only skill needed under the watchful eye of a midwife was to make sure that I didn't let the baby hit the floor!

Things changed by the time I came back as a fourth year medical student. I had gained more knowledge and some experience. The few nurses made rounds on the wards most days, while doctors saw the most problematic patients and did surgeries. When I arrived, I made rounds with one of the doctors on the men's and women's medical wards. He tried to visit those patients once a week. When we finished seeing the forty patients, he informed me that these would be my wards, showed me where the medical library was, and told me to feel free to seek him out with any questions.

The authors of this article would frown on that since I obviously lacked experience in "recognizing serious or unfamiliar conditions" and "performing particular procedures." They would also be concerned that I had inflated ideas about the value of my skills and lacked knowledge to work in a "limited laboratory" environment. They would also point out that I was disadvantaged by language, cultural, and other barriers. I'm sure they would have thought I was given responsibilities beyond my capability. In fact, most of the article has this tone. They admit that being thrust into these situations "can be exciting," but also say that "it can result in considerable stress and guilt in actions taken." The authors warn that trainees can get sick or be involved in accidents.

They point out that local staff and host institutions may have issues as well. They can neglect patients because they are spending time with visiting students or residents. It takes time to secure translators, provide orientation, and supervise. It may cost too much to provide food, lodging, and transport. Visiting students may spend too much time experiencing their exotic locations as tourists and not enough on their duties.

If you have been overseas long and hosted students, residents, and graduate doctors, you probably could go through those problems and attach a visitor's name to each problem they discussed! I certainly can from the hundreds of visiting staff during my time overseas.

Unfortunately, the article is too negative by not giving full value to the benefits of visiting staff, and it doesn't offer solutions or principles to guide institutions in these matters. Instead, they call for more research to address the problems discussed.

I guess we should not be surprised since secular institutions are relatively new to the issues raised in short-term service, whereas mission facilities have been providing these opportunities for forty to fifty years.

Here are some of the principles I employed in dealing with more than fifty short-term workers each year when I was overseas. Some will be a review for you and others may give you some new ideas.

Training Involves Greater Patient Risk
We are in agreement that we want to do the best we can to ensure competent and safe healthcare for our patients; yet, that understanding has to include both a short- and long-term view. Training new doctors and nurses always involves some risk for patients. We allow it because we will have less competent doctors in the future if we don't.

As I work with thousands of students in my role at CMDA, I sense the pendulum in the U.S. has swung too far over to the side of safety. Students don't have the procedural experience or the training in patient care that they need to be competently trained. More and more is done with "standardized patients" (actors) in role play situations and procedures are done with simulators. Some of these and other methods have their place, but an overemphasis on this versus actual patient care makes an inferior physician. It is one reason students are so eager to work overseas.

Where You Are is Not the U.S.
Transplanting what is the norm in the states to your mission facility won't work. It would have been better when I was a student if the long-term missionary doctor could make rounds on every patient. He couldn't. The missionary nurse with no formal diagnostic training couldn't see everyone. If she did, she wouldn't have time to improve the inadequate nursing services our patients experienced. Yes, I wasn't ideal. Yes, I was stretched and scared to death, but I did see every patient every day. I read, learned, asked questions, got consults, and learned procedures. Was I as good as the missionary doctor? No, but I would estimate the patients overall were better off just because they got more attention. I was the best available.

Build Good Systems
Take the time to create successful orientation for short-termers. Put up the appropriate fences for them to work within based on your patient load and the number of trained staff you have to meet them. Provide the best clinical supervision and training possible in your ministry while realizing it may fall far short of the ideal.

Improve
You have a moral obligation to make things better than they are. Usually the biggest issue is not enough physicians and nurses. Investing your time in visitors is your best hope of getting new staff to join you. As they come, move the fences to the appropriate place. Use these new people and newly developed methods to make your orientation, training, and mentoring better. Wherever possible, let visiting staff be part of what you are doing. Much more than new skills or knowledge is then transmitted. You will instill values, behavior, and beliefs into those following you around.

Address Outliers Quickly and Appropriately
With the checks and balances you put in place, you should be able to see who is breaking down the fences and straying. Rope them in quickly. Bring them back inside the fences, admonish them, and watch them more closely. Deepen your relationship with them. If they continue to stray, don't hesitate to throw them off the ranch.

It's More Than Medicine
Sometimes visitors can be more trouble than they are worth. Make sure you require them to stay long enough to give you some return on your investment as they gain knowledge and abilities and truly can help carry your load. But the bottom line to remember is this: your visitors are part of your mission field. For most, spending time working with you will have a profound and lasting effect on them as they draw closer to Christ and become more compassionate whether they practice overseas or not.

CHAPTER 8
THE NOBLE PURSUIT OF MEDICINE

*"*Is medicine a noble profession?" I continued. "What do you think?" he once again fired back. I waited. "No, it is not," he finally answered." - Dr. Sanjay Gupta interviewing Jack Kevorkian

If Jack had answered the question, "is medicine noble," instead of "is medicine a noble profession," I would have agreed with him. At best, Jack Kevorkian had a severely corrupted view on being a medical professional. We could easily argue he made no "profession" at all in the traditional Hippocratic tradition.

But back to the question, "Is medicine noble within itself?"

I think we would all agree that there is "good" medicine and "bad" medicine. A traditional medicine man in Africa, who we used to call a "witch doctor," will make dozens of small cuts over a painful area to release the evil spirits he believes is causing the disease. He will then rub a mixture of charcoal and herbs into the bleeding wounds to keep the evil spirits from returning. The end result is at best a placebo effect, but more likely only a diagnostic aid to the missionary doctor when the patient arrives at the hospital. You don't have to ask where it hurts but just find the mixture of old and fresh scars! I don't think you or I would call that form of "medicine" noble.

In the United States, we are increasingly returning to this same type of "medicine" practiced in Africa. I recently ran across an advertisement for Professor Vicki Noble who is described as a "feminist shamanic healer, independent scholar, author, and wisdom teacher" at Energy Medicine University. The advertisement promoted using her new version of tarot cards in diagnosing disease. This and other forms of alternative treatments such as therapeutic touch or homeopathy are more like traditional African medicine than a healthcare based on any scientifically proven benefits.

Sometimes such interventions may not be physically harmful, but instead can promote alternate spiritual belief systems or delay needed treatments until it is too late. Some of these practices have found fertile ground among Christians because they already believe in things that cannot be proven by the scientific method. You may have experienced these phenomena as I have, and I frequently hear a church member tout the many miraculous results of using colloidal silver.

But let's go deeper than this. The nobility of medicine does not lie simply on whether it is scientific or not, whether it is based on provable facts, and whether this knowledge is applied rightly. If so, our patients will be better off as soon as our examination rooms are occupied by Watson, the super computer that defeated the smartest "Jeopardy" contestants. No, the word noble carries the much richer meaning of "principled, moral, and virtuous."

Based on that definition, it is arguable that medicine is not noble within itself even in the classrooms and wards of our most prestigious hospitals. In these hospitals, medicine is increasingly regarded as a moral-neutral activity stripped of all values. It is simply the proper application of science, technology, and skill. There are no moral goals or required virtues. Doctors and nurses are simply technological experts, good "body mechanics" offering a quality service. The health professional's character, moral goals, and ethical outlook are inconsequential; these traits are considered private and personal issues. To demonstrate or share these personal characteristics imposes those views on others, making the healthcare provider guilty of "moral malpractice."

Medicine practiced in this manner is not noble. It is simply the amoral application of knowledge. The patient-doctor relationship is simply a contractual agreement between two parties governed by the preferences of the client. The "provider" is indentured to the "healthcare consumer" and has an obligation to fulfill the patient's whims within the boundaries of scientific standards. Serving personal autonomy is paramount to ensuring the healthcare consumer is satisfied.

In this prevalent view of medicine, the healthcare provider's actions are governed by law, government regulations, and pseudo-government professional standards. Doctors, nurses, and other healthcare personnel are expected to conform to these policies and penalized if they don't follow the rules. When healthcare lacks internalized standards, external controls of penalties and rewards are applied.

Though medicine is not noble within itself, I do believe there is a noble pursuit of medicine. It is based on the three "Cs"—convictions, character, and conduct. I don't have enough space or time to fully articulate all that the three "Cs" encompass, but let me give you a few examples.

The First C - Convictions
One core conviction is accountability. Remember Hwang Woo-Suk, the Korean scientist who fraudulently claimed he had successfully cloned human embryos? He maintained that deception for some time. After his duplicity was exposed, researchers rallied and demanded to know why the scientific community had not enforced accountability. That question is based on a faulty assumption. The truth is you can't achieve integrity through the regulations of the scientific community, and you achieve even less through the medical profession. Why? Because the doctor-patient relationship is too private and is protected from outside scrutiny. The doctor can easily falsify his records if he so desires as demonstrated by a news report on Dr. Kermit Gosnell, the infamous West Philadelphia abortionist. As *CBS.com* reported:

> *Dr. Kermit Gosnell, 69, faces eight counts of murder in the death of a woman following a botched abortion at his office, along with the deaths of seven other babies who, prosecutors allege, were born alive following illegal late-term abortions and then were killed by severing their spinal cords with a pair of scissors ... Gosnell is suspected of killing hundreds of living babies over the course of his 30-year practice. However, he is not charged because the records do not exist.*

Unfortunately, secularists assume what Johann Wolfgang von Goethe says is true, "As soon as you trust yourself, you will know how to live." I say that is rubbish! This statement completely ignores the sinful nature of every man or woman. That is why the firm conviction that you are answerable to a higher power who knows all, sees all, and even knows the motives in your heart is a foundational conviction that must be in place to ensure the noble pursuit of medicine. Though he was not a Christian, Hippocrates understood this. The Hippocratic oath states:

> *I swear by Apollo the healer, Asclepius, Hygeia and Panacea and I take to witness all the gods, all the goddesses, to keep according to my ability and my judgment, the following Oath and agreement ... If I fulfill this oath and do not violate it, may it be granted to me to enjoy life and art, being honored with fame among all men for all time to come; if I transgress it and swear falsely, may the opposite of all this be my lot.*

In its ancient form, the Hippocratic oath stands before higher beings and invites punishment from them if the practitioner does not adhere to the oath. To ensure virtue in the practice of medicine, the practitioner must be accountable. As Christians, we are held accountable to God Himself who knows our thoughts and motives.

The second conviction necessary for medicine to be a noble pursuit is a belief in human dignity, the belief that humans are worthy of the highest level of respect simply because they are human beings. Human dignity is not based on capabilities such as rational attributes like self-awareness, the ability to reason, or the ability to interact with the environment. Nor is it based on sentience—the fact that the human being is conscious and has the ability to feel pain, pleasure, or emotions. The source of human value is that we are valuable to God who designed us, who placed us on earth, and who gives us worth. Thus human dignity cannot be bestowed or taken away.

Regardless of an individual's religious persuasion or the lack of any persuasion at all, a belief in an innate human dignity is the only real position that allows our society to function and for people to live without fear. Otherwise who is protected, who is killed, who is valued, and who is discarded is determined only by those who have power.

For medicine to be a noble pursuit, the healthcare professional must also profess the conviction that there are things each professional ought to do and ought not to do. Our post-modern age says that is not the case. Objective moral truth is an illusion. At best, right and wrong are based on circumstances or cultural biases.

Some go further and maintain that right and wrong are just determined by majority rule. A post graduate student challenged me with this after I spoke at a medical school in Chicago. I responded, "Then the terrible medical experimentation sanctioned by Hitler in the concentration camps was right since a majority of people in Germany during World War II supported him and his views?" The student responded, "Of course."

This view that "might makes right" is chilling.

For medicine to be a noble pursuit, there must be a conviction by the professional that some things are morally wrong; not because of changeable codes, regulations, or laws, but because they are objectively wrong for everyone at all times.

It is wrong to take sexual advantage of a patient. It is wrong to betray a patient's confidence. It is wrong to neglect a patient's need for treatment. It is wrong to harm the patient by over-medicating. It is wrong to do harmful human research. It is wrong to prescribe a more expensive drug because the drug representative selling that drug took you out to dinner last night. It is wrong to kill your patient. The conviction of objective moral truth is essential to the noble practice of medicine.

The Second C - Character
For the pursuit of medicine to be noble, it is not enough to have convictions or beliefs. The practitioner must have a virtuous character, the second C.

The following virtues of the medical practitioner have been well articulated by Edmund D. Pellegrino and David C. Thomasma in *The Virtues of Medical Practice*.

- Trustworthiness
- Compassion
- Prognosis (practical wisdom)
- Justice

- Fortitude
- Temperance
- Integrity
- Self-Effacement
- Faith
- Hope
- Charity

Healthcare professionals face an ever expanding medical knowledge, the motivation of money, their own personal tiredness, insurance company directives, time limitations, government intrusion into the doctor/patient relationship, and a host of other factors. The best insurance the clinician will act for the patient's good despite these extensive influences is that the healthcare professional is inherently good. No code or conviction can cover all contingencies. There are too many variables in the practice of medicine.

Let's focus on just a few of the character qualities most essential in the noble pursuit of medicine.

In a 2010 Gallup poll, survey takers were asked to "tell me how you would rate the honesty and ethical standards of people in these different fields." The highest trust was put in nurses (81 percent), military officers (73 percent), and pharmacists (71 percent). Physicians dropped to 66 percent, followed by police officers (57 percent), and clergy (53 percent). The three last places were congressmen (9 percent), used car salesmen (7 percent), and lobbyists (7 percent).

As a physician, I'm concerned that only two out of every three potential patients find us to be honest and ethical, because the foundation of the doctor-patient relationship is trust. If doctors continue to not be considered trustworthy, our medical system will be fatally wounded. That is one of the reasons I fight so hard against the legalization of physician-assisted suicide. You cannot trust a doctor who can both cure you and kill you. We've seen that in the Netherlands where fearful elderly citizens carry cards saying, "Please don't euthanize me," out of fear a doctor will kill them if they are seriously ill and taken to a hospital.

Another essential characteristic is reliability. Reliability is the willingness to be there for your patients just like in the marriage covenant "in sickness and in health." It is ironic that today's younger physicians idealize a practice style of very limited availability—no night call, no weekends, etc.—at the same time when patients are demanding more availability. Patients want to be able to tweet or post a status update with their questions and their concerns to their doctor at any time. We have gained more convenience with same-day appointments, walk-in clinics, and 24/7 emergency rooms; at the same time, you lose the personal relationship you would normally encounter when seeing a doctor who knows you.

I'm not advocating a 24/7 medical practice without boundaries, but noble medicine is not a "9 to 5" job. I fear the pendulum is swinging too far from unlimited commitment to unreliableness in the U.S.

Another essential characteristic in the noble pursuit of medicine is that the healthcare professional must be responsible and conscientious. When patients put their health and even their lives into your hands, they want someone who is obsessive-compulsive and will pay attention to even the smallest details.

Dr. Sam Molind, the oral surgeon who previously led CMDA's Global Health Outreach, related a story to me of his work in Hanoi, Vietnam, where he has traveled to train doctors and residents annually for more than fifteen years. The chair of oral surgery at the medical school tapped him on the shoulder as he was scrubbing for a case and asked, "Are you a Christian?" Not knowing his motives, Sam said, "Why do you ask?"

The chair said, "I've noticed you always talk to the patient's family before and after a surgery. We only talk to the family if there are unexpected problems. We go home on weekends and don't come into the hospital to even see our post-op patients, but you come in every single day and check on each one. Your conscientiousness makes me think you may be a Christian." Sam told the chair that he was a Christian, and the chair went on to say, "We want to train our doctors to be like you."

Another noble principle of medicine is truthfulness. When a physician or nurse communicates with patients, honesty fosters confidence and shows respect. Truthfulness is a prerequisite to engender trust. If a patient discovers or perceives a lack of honesty and candor by the physician, trust is destroyed.

In 1961, only 10 percent of physicians surveyed believed it was correct to tell a patient of a fatal cancer diagnosis. By 1979, 97 percent felt that such disclosure was correct. Without being told their diagnosis, prognosis, and treatment options, patients cannot fully participate in their own healthcare decision-making. Of course, there can be some inconsequential information that does not need to be shared and some information that needs to be shared in a sensitive and tactful way.

Can being truthful be harmful at times? Rarely, and then it is often due to the patient's culture. If the physician has some compelling reason to think that disclosure would create a real and predictable harmful effect on the patient, it may be justified to withhold truthful information. For example, sharing a terminal diagnosis with a suicidal patient may cause that patient to act upon impulse.

At times, a patient may request to not be informed but rather have the information be discussed with his or her family. Complete disclosure may also be hampered by the patient's mental capacity to understand and process the doctor's information.

No list of the essential character traits healthcare professionals must demonstrate to nobly pursue medicine would be complete without mentioning competence. Competence is a blend of knowledge and experience that leads to good judgment, what many of us would call wisdom.

Competence is not just knowledge. All of us know healthcare professionals who have near photographic memories but lack the common sense and insight to apply that knowledge. Having competence requires the virtues of self-discipline to continually learn. Unfortunately, educational institutions and professional bodies increasingly use coercion to persuade professionals to maintain competency with ever-increasing certification and recertification requirements. It would seem better to inspire continual learning through the character virtue of self-discipline.

The Final C – Conduct
For medicine to be a noble pursuit, conviction and character must also engender right conduct. For example, patients desire healthcare professionals to demonstrate compassion. It is not sufficient to be technically fit, diagnose rare diseases, or prescribe the correct treatments. We must show kindness, personal warmth, empathy, and care for each patient's desires and needs. We may take exams to prove technical competence, but the qualities of compassion are not easily measured. That does not mean they are not important. We must take that imaginative leap into our patients' shoes. As author Joseph Campbell says, "Compassion is suffering with the patient."

When I was serving in Kenya, I was asked to speak at a CMDE meeting in Malaysia. On my way home I developed a severe headache, fever, and muscle aches; I thought I had resistant malaria since I had been taking prophylaxis. I ended up in an emergency room in Bangkok with a group of interns and an standing attending at the end of my stretcher discussing my case in a language I couldn't understand. An intern returned to tell me in halting English, "You okay. No malaria." I make it back to Kenya only to be diagnosed with viral meningitis.

In addition to recovering physically, I also developed better compassion towards my patients. I too had stood at the end of their beds discussing them in a language they didn't understand. It is helpful for healthcare professionals to suffer disease to enable them to appreciate what it feels like to be the patient. We then become better in responding to our patients with compassion.

The Greek tragedies and comedies were morality plays teaching important principles. The comedies taught not to descend into hubris and not to take yourself too seriously. Tragedies told the audience that there were consequences for wrong actions and outlined important ethical principles to be adhered to by the audience.

The Greek playwright Sophocles told the story of Philoctetes who is abandoned by his fellow sailors on a desolate island because of his severe wounds. They couldn't tolerate his noisy suffering any longer. Philoctetes speaks of his exile and gives us insight into the suffering of our patients who each occupy their own "island" of suffering, cut off from the life and friends they know. He says,

> ...let me tell you of this island. No one comes here willingly. There is no anchorage here, nor any place to land, profit in trade, and be received.

In the play, a young man happens on the island and tries to end the wounded warrior's exile. The young man earns Philoctetes' trust and gratitude by staying with him through a severe time of pain and then unconsciousness. When he wakes up, Philoctetes marvels that the young man has not abandoned him in his suffering. He says,

> ...blessed is a friend's protection. These things are beyond my wildest hopes, that you would pity me and care for my sorrows, that you would remain by me and endure my woes.

Like the young man, each of us needs to visit our patients' islands and learn something from their lonely exile. Trust and a greater understanding will grow out of that shared experience.

The last conduct I want to mention is the practice of altruism, an unselfish concern for the welfare of others. The nobleness of the pursuit of medicine is often best demonstrated by our care for the poor and powerless. Like the Good Samaritan, healthcare professionals should be willing to give their expertise, time, and money to care for those in need, even to the point of putting themselves at risk. As our accountability agent, God didn't call us to safety, security, or comfort. He called us to lay down our lives for others.

Maybe that is why He attached good physiological consequences to practicing altruism. Studies clearly show that altruistic behavior decreases stress, increases immunity, relieves pain, improves emotional health, decreases anxiety, relieves depression, increases longevity, and improves social interaction. Interestingly, these health benefits are tied to giving of yourself. You don't get them by giving your money alone.

I've experienced this firsthand. When I served as a missionary doctor, we had many "short-termers," physicians and dentists who traveled to Kenya to help us for a month. Usually around the end of their first week, one of them would say something like this, "Dave, I'm having a wonderful time." To which I would usually reply, "Really? You haven't worked this hard since your internship." Then they would say, "Yes, but I'm not worrying about getting paid. I'm not worrying about getting sued. Patients so appreciate what I'm doing for them and I'm saving lives every day! Being here brings back to me all the reasons I went into medicine in the first place."

Many of these doctors returned again and again. I called them "short-term mission junkies" who came back again and again to get their "helper's high" fix, or what Dr. John Patrick calls, "Level II Happiness."

The Noble in Medicine
Medicine is not inherently noble within itself. The nobility of medicine resides in that constant striving of the individual practitioner who has foundational convictions but also pursues honorable character and conduct.

I hope you have the opportunity to meet just one or two magnificent "nobles" of the healthcare profession. They are honorable, virtuous, and self-sacrificing. They are so magnetic that there is healing in their very presence.

Two nobles immediately come to my mind.

I can still remember spending an hour and a half driving Dr. Paul Brand to the airport after he spoke at a CMDA conference. It was an unforgettable conversation as he inspired and encouraged me. He shared stories and insights into God's Word that probed my mind and heart while ministering to me. I didn't want him to get out of the car at the airport.

I knew Dr. Steury the best. I talk about him throughout this book because he had such a profound impact upon my career and my life. He was my friend, father figure, mentor, teacher, and example during the eleven years I worked at Tenwek. He knew more than any doctor I have ever worked with, but he wrapped his competence in a cloak of humility. He knew God had called him to serve the Kipsigis people, and he treated his patients like royalty. As a physician, he brought more than just healing for the bodies that would ultimately die. He brought the healing of the gospel for their souls that would live forever.

His character was above approach and he lived a life of self-sacrifice. During his first ten years in Kenya, he was on call 24/7. Nothing was too big or too small for him to do in order to serve others. He would resect a black swollen sigmoid volvulus that smelled so bad it would gag a maggot, and then he would help the mechanic get the hospital generator going again. He was loved and venerated by all who knew him. Multitudes attended his memorial services; presidents called him friend; people wanted to just be in his presence.

If Ernie was alive, he would not see himself as I've described him. He would in no way think he had accomplished the noble practice of medicine. For him, carrying out his profession at the highest level and serving his Lord was simply his daily pursuit.

Don't you want to be like that? I do. I want to be like a drop of water that hits the water and sends ripples of God's grace into other people's lives. What a noble pursuit!

PART 3
PLANNING AND ADMINISTRATION

CHAPTER 9
BOARDS THAT WORK

Boards can make or break missionary medical ministry. We are going to look at board structure and function as well as the important relationship between governance and administration. What principles make it work well? What is likely to cause a tumultuous relationship that hampers the mission of the organization? Though it is often the CEO of the medical ministry who deals with the board, its decisions impact everyone in the mission healthcare system.

Though the focus will be on the medical system, the ideas can help you improve the structure and governance capabilities of other organizations. Missionary doctors and other healthcare personnel often serve on a variety of governance groups within their mission systems. For example, I was on the board of the Kenya Highlands University and served on the mission "field committee" that established policies. Other governance groups need to apply the same principles and you may be in a position to help do that.

Let's start with the board makeup. Many mission hospitals and/or healthcare projects have been completely turned over to the church so their governing bodies are made up of only pastors. In most instances, that doesn't work well. Why? Because the average pastor does not have the experience or training to understand the complex issues of healthcare.

Should you have pastors on the board? Of course! Your medical outreach is not just about medicine. It is also about evangelism of patients, counseling, and hopefully church planting. You need the perspective and experience of pastors. They are the communication mode for joint projects and their expertise is invaluable. They open the church network for you so their partnership is invaluable.

But a governance board should have a variety of skill sets represented on it. Ideally, you should have a board member with expertise and experience in each aspect of your outreach. You need people who know medicine, people who know the church, people who are familiar with education if you have training schools, etc. You may need board members with government contacts, marketing experience, or other knowledge.

What if your board is already made up of only pastors? If you can't change that to a broader representation, then look for church leaders with expertise and experience beyond pastoring. CMDA's board is totally made up of doctors. We are locked into this as a membership organization, but the board actively looks for doctors who have media, public policy, missions, evangelism, and other expertise so that every aspect of CMDA's ministry has a board member who can open networks and help the board understand issues that arise.

Major stakeholders should also be represented on your governing body. At Tenwek, the board was made up of one-third church leaders, one-third missionaries, and one-third community and government leaders. It was a healthy balance of stakeholders who acted as checks and balances. Though they never actually wanted to, the group of church leaders was unable to drain money from the hospital for church projects. The group of government leaders was unable to dominate the board for political gain. Not having the missionaries in the majority was good public relations in the community, yet it still let them have input into the decisions made. Every group of stakeholders "owned" the hospital because they were involved through their representatives in running it.

An added bonus was that we could emphasize different "ownership" to the varied potential support groups. If we were having a "harambee" to raise funds for the hospital in the community, we could genuinely emphasize that Tenwek was "their hospital." When we were approaching para-government organizations for project funding, we would emphasize that the hospital was run by an independent board and not a denomination. When approaching churches or Christian foundations, we would emphasize that Tenwek was a mission hospital and include involvement of the church and mission in its governance. Practically and conceptually, the various stakeholder representations helped us carry out our mission.

How should trustees or board members be selected? It is important that the board have a significant say in the selection process to ensure that the types of board members needed are obtained. That doesn't mean the stakeholders have no say, but the ball should not totally be in their court. If it is, the church will often pick who has the time, who lives close by, or who holds a certain office with little regard for whether that person has the basic skills and the type of expertise needed. One way to handle this is to have a committee of the board that analyzes the level of expertise currently on the board and puts together a profile of the type of board members needed. That profile can then be given to the stakeholder groups to fill the allotted slots. Even better is to have the board chair meet with church, government, or community leaders to discuss the profiles needed and jointly select candidates. The full board should then have the final approval of candidates.

One helpful planning aid is to create a grid with the present board members listed down one side and the areas of expertise needed listed down the other side. Then fill in the grid to see what areas are covered and which areas of knowledge or experience lack representation.

How often should the board meet? Usually two or three meetings per year are sufficient, though circumstances may require otherwise. Often a board meeting that lasts one or two days is more productive than shorter, more frequent meetings. It takes time to get into the governance groove, get caught up on reports, and have discussion.

What is the board's job? This is where many organizations get into trouble with the board doing the administration's job or vice versa. A few decades ago when CMDA was having financial problems, the board had meetings that lasted three to four days and spent time making decisions such as whether or not to buy a new copier. Doctors are used to solving problems, so they were doing the administration's job.

A board's job description is actually rather short.

1. Supervision – The board has the responsibility to hire, supervise, evaluate, and fire the organization's highest-level employee, such as the CEO or hospital administrator.
2. Fiscal Responsibility – The board has the responsibility to ensure the financial integrity of the organization. It approves the budget, monitors the accounting, selects the auditor, approves the audit, and makes sure adequate safeguards are in place.
3. Strategic Planning – The board sets the vision, mission, values, and major goals of the organization. It monitors adherence to the vision, mission, and goals of the organization and evaluates whether the goals of the organization are being accomplished.
4. Policy – The board defines the major policies that govern the work. In other words, the trustees set the fences within which the executive officer and the staff can operate.
5. Representation – The board communicates and listens to key constituents to remain informed and make sure the organization is accomplishing its purpose.
6. Self-Evaluation and Improvement – The board evaluates itself and brings in people to train it to do a better job.

How does this differ from the staff's and CEO's jobs? The board decides what needs to be done in broad terms by establishing major goals. For example, the board may set a goal of having 85 percent immunization in your service area. The CEO then decides how to accomplish the established goals. What staff, money, facilities, and organization are needed? What programs or services need to be offered to reach the goal set?

The board sets the boundaries by establishing policies the staff may function within, and the CEO is free to make all the decisions if he/she stays inside the boundaries. As part of the financial boundaries, the board policies may include statements such as:

1. The health system is expected to have a positive balance sheet at the end of the year.
2. The CEO will ensure that staff members are paid salary levels

established by the government health system for health workers.
3. The health system will not borrow money without board approval.
4. The administration will establish adequate financial safeguards to prevent embezzlement.
5. The organization will keep three-months cash reserves.

To ensure the hospital stays within these boundaries, the CEO will then work with the administration to establish subsidiary policies and procedures which might include more check signers for larger checks, cross checks of receipts each day, etc.

Using distinct complementary roles applies to other areas as well. The board may set the goal of increasing your catchment size by 20 percent. The CEO then decides whether or not to raise funds, hire staff, and build dispensaries or health centers to reach the goal while still remaining within the stipulated financial boundaries.

It often takes reminders to make sure the trustees or administration don't stray into others' areas of responsibility. Let me give you an example. A few years ago, CMDA's board established an ad hoc committee of dentists to advise the board on reaching out to dentists. In his report to the board, the committee chair recommended that a dental director be hired to oversee this area.

Not a bad idea, but I had to say, "Wait a minute. Whether we hire a dental director or not is my job, not yours. You can set a goal of doubling our dental membership or reaching out to 20 percent more dental campuses, but how we accomplish the goal is my job."

The administration is often involved in proposing goals and even drawing up draft policies, but the board makes the final decisions. The board formulates policies and determines goals, but the CEO and administration are in charge of implementation needed to reach those goals.

The board is also responsible for monitoring to ensure that policies are adhered to and that goals are met. This should happen at least yearly if not at every meeting.

What principles make a board efficient?

1. Not too large or too small. If the board is too small, there are not enough people to get the work done. If it is too large, it becomes unwieldy and too hard to get decisions made. Boards of ten to twenty people seem to work well.
2. Board Standing Committees. The board should be divided into three subcommittees that meet and do their work at the beginning of each board meeting. Usually there is a finance committee, a strategic planning/monitoring committee, and a board affairs committee. Each committee has a chair selected by the board chairman, as well as someone from the administration who meets with the committee. For example, the CEO may meet with the strategic planning committee and the chief financial officer may meet with the finance committee. The committees meet for a half-day to plan and monitor. They then bring their monitoring reports to the full board and make resolutions for policies and goals that the board approves. This speeds decision-making and lets the board do its work in less time.
3. It is good to make annual calendars for each committee to create consistency in its projects. For example, the board affairs committee may formulate a list of potential trustees at its fall meeting each year and prioritize that list. At the winter meeting, they review the resumes of those who agreed to serve and recommend names to the board. The board decides to invite the candidates to the spring meeting and make a decision at the end of the board meeting. As another example, the finance committee may always examine the audit in the fall and ask for a report on insurance coverage for your facility at every winter meeting.
4. Have a timed agenda for each meeting. The chair estimates how long each item will take and then keeps the board meeting moving. The agenda and support materials—resolutions, background information, etc.—should be circulated to the trustees a couple of weeks prior to the meeting for review.
5. Keep useful minutes. Minutes should be complete and easily referenced. I recommend numbering the minutes sequentially during the calendar year. Out to the side of a minute might be "15/09/12" showing that it is the fifteenth item addressed

at the September 2012 board meeting. Each motion should be done in bold so they can be easily pulled out. I also suggest underlining action items such as the "CEO will bring a report on outpatient utilization to the next meeting." The board secretary can easily pull these out and make a list of each person's tasks for the next meeting.

The board members wear three hats. The "Governance Hat" is only worn in a properly called meeting with a quorum. This is the legal authority hat and it is only worn in the group, never when working alone. In other words, the board member has no authority over the administration except when they are acting as part of the board group. The "Volunteer Hat" goes on when the trustee leaves the board meeting. It carries no authority but is worn by trustees while fundraising, advising, or helping the staff in some other way. When helping the staff, they are under the supervision of the staff.

The "Implementer Hat" has limited authority specifically given to the trustee by the board as a whole. It is seldom worn since the administration normally implements tasks. The only time it is worn is when the board or CEO gives a board member authority to carry out a specific task such as collecting information or fact-finding. This hat is taken off once the job is complete.

The chair of the board leads the meetings and communicates decisions of the board to the CEO. This person also interprets the board's decisions if they are not understood by the administrative team. The chair also encourages and helps the CEO accomplish the mission. The chair carries no authority to make individual decisions or impose his/her will on the administration.

The CEO should have a formal evaluation by the board each year. My evaluation is at the winter board meeting. I do a written self-assessment of how well I've met the board's goals and discuss my relationship with the board, my needs, concerns, etc. How can I improve? What continuing education have I done and what is needed? Then I meet for discussion and assessment with the chair and vice chair who reviewed my evaluation. They then carry a report to the entire board to decide whether I continue in my role and what admonishment or encouragement I need.

That concept of annual evaluations brings up other important items. At every board meeting, the board should do two things. One is a self-evaluation. What worked well? How could they have done better? How did the logistics work? It doesn't take long, but this introspective analysis is very valuable and should be on the agenda.

Secondly, the board should have executive session. At the end of the board meeting, all staff in attendance should be excused except for the CEO. The CEO can bring any concerns to the board for discussion and the board can ask any questions they may have. The CEO is then excused while his or her performance is discussed privately. Why is this so important? If this is not done, board business begins to happen outside the board meeting because trustees aren't at liberty to have a private discussion. Doing business outside the board meeting leads to politicking by groups within the board which is very destructive. Board business should only be done in the board meeting. It is also important to keep short accounts and not let things build up if there are problems with the CEO. Executive session minutes are kept separate from the circulated minutes. The chair acts as the spokesperson to the CEO. Having an executive session at every meeting ensures that they are not done just when there is a crisis. Often they are very short but still important.

Each new board member should be trained. We currently complete this training prior to a new member's first board meeting. A present trustee should also be appointed to act as a mentor to the new member. The two then sit together at the meetings to allow the mentor to explain issues and procedures. New board members should be encouraged to participate from day one. It is helpful to have a board profile section in your board manual with information about each board member to facilitate relationship building. One way to recruit and utilize board members well is to have a board member job description. That makes the board's expectation for members clear.

Each year, CMDA trustees sign two documents. One is an affirmation that they are still in agreement with CMDA's statement of faith, purposes, and goals. It also states they are still committed to support CMDA with their prayers, time, expertise, and finances. The second document is a potential "conflict of interest" document meant to reveal their relationships with other organizations that CMDA may deal with. Conflicts of interest are normal, but should be revealed if other relationships can influence decisions the trustee makes on the board.

Lastly, the board polices should be gathered into one document that is updated at every meeting. If not, decisions made years ago might be lost or forgotten. Board-standing policies detail governance policies, the CEO-board parameters, and boundaries that have been set. At each board meeting, policies are added, deleted, or modified so this is a living document.

As you can see from this chapter, there is a large amount of details to good governance. Though we have just done an overview, there are great printed resources on non-profit boards. I recommend the *Non-profit Board Answer Book: Practical Guidelines for Board Members and Chief Executives* by Robert C. Andringa and Ted Engstrom, available at *www.amazon.com*.

This brings me to my last recommendation. The best investment you can make is to have an outside person come in and train your board. I did that when I arrived at CMDA and it has borne huge dividends. In fact, we do it every four years because of our board turnover. As the CEO, it is difficult to tell the board what they need to do, but an outside expert carries lots of clout.

Building a strong governance foundation is the first key to a strong organization.

CHAPTER 10
THE CEO

Outstanding administration has to be built on the foundation of good governance, a concept we just addressed. We will begin to discuss the structure and function of the administrative side of the equation. Your goal is to create a well-lubricated, smooth running operation so you can accomplish the mission God has called you to.

Administrative principles can be learned the easy way or the hard way. You can read, observe, and be mentored, or you can learn from your mistakes. I confess, I have had lessons from both sources, but I hope to help you learn most of yours the easy way.

The first principle is that someone has to be in charge. Committees and teams have their place in administration, but usually do a poor job in running an institution if they are the final authority. Decisions tend to drift to the lowest common denominator. Committees play it safe and don't take risks or develop bold initiatives. It is impossible for the board to hold a committee accountable or really supervise its members. Committee members often represent different constituencies in your institution and see issues from their group's perspective. Without a final authority to serve as a referee, you can rapidly develop the "silo" effect. Each department or division walls itself off from others and seeks only its own good.

The second principle is to pick the right person to be in charge. The board selects and manages the administrator or the CEO. This person holds the complete authority and responsibilities for running the medical outreach. This individual carries out the policies and directs the ministry in order to reach the goals of the board.

Who should this person be? I would look for the following characteristics. Other things could be added to this list, but these five areas are the most critical in my experience.

1. Vision – Without a vision, the people perish and so does the medical mission. A visionary sees further down the path than others do. He or she sees the big picture of where the institution is and where it needs to go. This person is driven by a vision to be an agent of change. Individuals with this drive are the ones with the ideas for new outreaches, new procedures, new policies, new personnel, and greater impact.
2. Organizational Skills – Too often visionaries have the vision, but lack the management skills to get it done. If the visionary CEO has a good chief operating officer (COO) with the skills to get it done, it can still work; however, in my experience, that luxury is unusual in mission facilities. In the mission facilities that excel, the leader has the organizational skills and self-discipline to get the job done when no one else is available to do it. Many barriers exist to offering good health and spiritual care in a mission facility. A great CEO cannot only see the destination, but also figures how to get there and takes the steps necessary to acclimate to the journey. This organizational person can organize people and resources to accomplish the vision.
3. Charisma – "The ability to inspire enthusiasm, interest, or affection in others by means of personal charm or influence." One of the nicest compliments I've ever received was from the president of CMDA the year I started. We were considering the bold step of moving from Dallas, Texas, to Bristol, Tennessee, and using donated space in a pharmaceutical company building. I was recruiting my team and asked Dr. Gene Rudd, who worked with me at Samaritan's Purse, to join us in Bristol for the visit. We had breakfast at a restaurant along with a great conversation. When Dr. Rudd stepped away to the restroom, the president turned to me and said in reference to Gene, "The best measure of a leader is the quality of people he or she attracts to work with them." That's so true. A good leader attracts good staff. A great leader attracts and develops leaders who make the job much easier. These types of leaders are able to get others enthused about their mission and

goals. That is what Dr. Steury did to me as a college student in 1972 when I spent time living in his home and following him around the hospital. When I returned home, it was with the goal to someday become half the medical missionary doctor that Ernie Steury was. He inspired me through medical school and residency, and his legacy still inspires me today.
4. Problem Solving Skills – Being a medical missionary means dealing with one problem after another. Worse than the clinical problems are the relational and logistical ones. It is tough when you live, work, worship, and vacation with the same people. Often mission life is a very socialistic enterprise. Though everyone is treated the same by the mission, their needs are not the same. Policies often don't apply well to those working night and day in medical institutions. Workloads are heavy, and your workload can increase to unbearable levels when someone takes vacation or is sick. Many missionaries live on compounds where the group decides how the new missionary's house will be built. I can still remember the discussion about whether the house we raised money to build would be the first one with more than one bathroom! All these things and more lead to interpersonal conflicts; if not dealt with, these conflicts cause heartache, bitterness, and broken relationships. The person in charge has to deal with these problems, as well as make sure electricity, water, penicillin, and money to pay the staff are readily available. You have to deal with church/mission conflicts, problems with the regulating authority, tensions between different ethnic groups working in the institution, and the list goes on. The CEO needs to be a good problem solver and needs to be ready to take the bull by the horns when problems arise.
5. Spiritual Maturity – The person at the top needs to be respected and inspired for spiritual leadership and maturity. If that individual doesn't have those characteristics, the mission will drift, the wrong type of people will be recruited, and the wrong solutions will be applied to problems. Medical missions is a spiritual warfare, and it is not for the ill equipped or faint of heart. You want a general who is living daily in the presence of the Commander-in-Chief.

Should this position be filled by a national or a missionary? A national should be your goal, but finding one with the essential skills and training is difficult. Often someone needs to be identified, mentored, sent for training, and moved up in the organization with greater responsibilities as progress is shown. Many mission groups fail to do this well, or suddenly decide to put a national in charge who doesn't have the personal characteristics, skills, or experience. That is a recipe for disaster.

The exact same thing often happens with a missionary leader. Often a good leader established the institution, but retires, gets sick, goes on extended home assignment, or passes away. The tendency is to then look around and see who among the present staff might be able to fit the position. Often that person lacks the whole package needed and doesn't have the relationships, reputation, language skills, experience, or maturity to do the job well. As a result, the institution languishes.

I believe mission organizations and institutional boards should be much more proactive. They should search for and recruit good leaders just as a secular organization does. They should have a succession plan in place years before it is needed so they can begin to prepare that person or persons for future roles. Mission organizations often wait until someone shows up at the door applying to be a missionary, and then they pray that individual will be just the person they need. Why not search for mature Christians who have already been successful? Look for individuals who might consider a second career overseas. Look for young people who were chief residents, president of their college classes, or hold accomplishments showing leadership skills. Approach them about considering mission service and begin mentoring them for the leadership. Identify people already on the mission field who have potential. What training and experience do they need? Who should mentor them? How should they progress through levels of responsibility before they are tapped for the big one?

I am amazed at how institutional boards and mission organizations are such poor stewards in this area. They place poorly prepared people as heads of large and complex organizations, and pray that God will make up for their lack of planning and initiative. The greatest need in medical missions today is great leaders. That is why the Center for Medical Missions exists to inspire and train leaders for every level needed to build God's kingdom through medical missions.

If you already are or likely will be the CEO of the institution, what are you doing to get prepared? What training, mentoring, or experience do you need? Where can you acquire that training? Have you sat down with your present leaders to discuss what needs to be done, and when and how it is going to be paid for? If they won't be proactive, you should be.

The bad news is that doctors often have little training or experience in leadership and administration. The good news is that they know how to assimilate and apply large amounts of information. They are quick learners. I believe a portion of each home assignment period should be set aside for training, and the most needed training is often in non-medical arenas.

If you are already a reluctant CEO, seek counsel on what you need to learn while also developing your skills to become good at what you are now doing. Read books, visit other successful institutions, find a mentor even if it is one by e-mail, ask questions, take a correspondence course, or even request to spend a number of months with a successful medical missionary leader to learn. It will be time well invested.

Let me throw out one more radical idea. If you can, consider a co-CEO relationship. You're probably saying, "Wait a minute, you said the board needs to hold one person accountable!" True, someone has to be in charge, so I'm not talking about structure, but practice. When I was at Tenwek, Dr. Steury and I had this type of relationship. Both of us had full knowledge of even the stickiest situations. We bounced ideas off each other, envisioned, and planned. We divided the CEO's workload. We had complete confidence in each other, didn't care who got the credit, and always backed each other's decisions. Dr. Steury was ultimately in charge, but he delegated most of the full weight of his authority to me as well. We did discuss the critical or important issues, but we simply handled many of the routine things. Some issues were important to tell the other about, and some were not. He was called the Executive Officer while I was the Medical Superintendent, but it was a co-CEO relationship.

I still use the same system at CMDA. Dr. Rudd is my "Associate Executive Director." We divide the supervision of senior staff. He handles the support areas—finance, personnel, IT, and membership services. I directly supervise the outward looking areas such as public policy, stewardship, missions, and campus ministries.

The beauty of the system is that we move faster and better toward our goals with two CEOs. Everyone knows that the buck stops with me, but Dr. Rudd speaks for me. We don't always make the same decisions in a situation, but we don't make a greater proportion of wrong ones. I'm completely loyal to him and him to me. We both know all the important stuff. We are not clones, but we both have all the abilities needed to lead the organization. He is better in some areas than I am, and I'm better in some areas than he is.

When the Christian Management Association and *Christianity Today* selected CMDA as the best Christian workplace a few years ago, this unique relationship and structure is what they featured in their article. It shouldn't be unique to CMDA. I know it can work in a mission facility and it can work across generational lines. Ernie was twenty years older than me, and he certainly didn't hand me a co-CEO relationship the first day. He let me learn the culture, language, and missionary medicine the first few years, then he handed me the community health program as a new endeavor to organize and lead. He didn't look over my shoulder, but was available for advice and input. I kept him informed. He increasingly kept me informed of what was going on with other projects and sought my advice. By his next furlough, I was the acting CEO.

We've spent time discussing the key leaders of each institution. Next, we turn our attention to creating the right structures while putting the right people in place and helping them be successful.

CHAPTER 11
SENIOR STAFF

At CMDA, we refer to the people at the next level as Senior Staff and they are the directors who lead their departments, but your nomenclature can be whatever fits your situation. In medical situations, it might be Matron, Nursing Director, Medical Superintendent, Administrator, etc. The term Senior Staff lets others know that these people report directly to the CEO.

Employees at this level need good leadership skills, but their primary roles are people management and administration. If they have visionary capabilities as well, it is a great bonus.

In my experience, the key to developing an effective and well-run organization is recruiting the right people. If you find them, your job will be much easier and your ministry will prosper, so it is crucial to find them.

The first step is to develop a job description. Define the purpose of the position in one to two sentences, then list the duties the person will be responsible to accomplish. Ideally, there should be no more than ten listed, so you may need to consolidate activities under broader headings. These two items, purpose and duties, constitute the first sections of a one-page job description. The last duty should always state, "Other duties as may be assigned by the CEO." This avoids staff members claiming something that you ask them to do is not in their job description.

The next two sections are short—"Responsible For" and "Responsible To." Obviously, senior staff members are responsible to the CEO, but may be responsible for a few to many people that they supervise. For a medical superintendent, a broad phrase such as "all medical personnel" may be used instead of listing each job title.

The last two sections are "Minimal Acceptable Qualifications" and "Additional Desirable Qualifications." The first of these contains a list of the training, experience, degrees, or abilities that are essential for the job. If I were appointing a medical superintendent, I would want to put on my minimal list items such as:

1. A personal relationship with Jesus Christ and an exemplary Christian witness
2. Compatible with the purposes and practices of the institution
3. Visionary leadership ability
4. Personnel and program management expertise
5. An MD degree
6. A high level of professional competence.

On my additional list, I might add:

1. Experience as a medical superintendent in a hospital
2. Second or third language fluency
3. Additional levels of training or certification
4. Miscellaneous

Get the idea? Also, job descriptions should have a small note at the bottom noting when the most recent revision took place, so you will recognize the latest version in your files. Job descriptions should be reviewed yearly. The advantage of developing a job description is that it requires you to carefully consider what the job entails and the kind of person you need to recruit. I always run a proposed job description by someone else to make sure I've thought of everything and then make sure I meet the criteria I've set as I recruit the person. Don't fudge on the minimal qualifications criteria or you will regret it. A job description can be circulated among your current staff to see if people would like to apply for the position, as well as given to prospective outside candidates.

A job description should be available for every position in your institution, but the CEO doesn't need to write each one. Ideally, job descriptions are written by the position's immediate supervisor, and copies should be in the hands of the administrator, the immediate supervisor, and the employee.

I always look first within the organization for an employee to fill a higher position. This lets staff know that good performance is rewarded with promotions and a higher salary. This is a powerful motivator to your current employees, but also provides great benefits to you as well. You already know the performance, personality, strengths, and weaknesses of your present staff members. You are not taking a shot in the dark by basing your decision on a resume and a brief interview from someone from outside the institution. Remember to set a deadline for present staff to apply by, and then go outside the organization to look for new people.

I remind myself often that I want to hire an "A" team. The tendency is to hire quickly to fill a much-needed position. When this is done, you often end up with "B" or "C" employees. What do I mean?

"A" employees are innovators and problem solvers. They take you to the next level. They are like a dovetail joint. They perfectly fit their positions as leaders and take their work arenas to higher planes of effectiveness. They often do their jobs better than their supervisors could. They are knowledgeable, organized, self-disciplined, and are leaders admired and followed by staff members. They are visionaries who can make their visions become reality.

"B" employees do a good job at their duties, but lack the vision to innovate and the skills and initiative to solve difficult people problems. These employees can grind the gears, but they don't pour oil in them and don't take the initiative to design a better machine through strategic planning and implementation. As the supervisor, you have to step in and complete that part of the job, pulling you away from your responsibilities. If you have lots of "B" employees, you don't have enough time to do this, problems multiply, or the organization fails to move forward. A "B" employee is an adequate manager, but lacks the leadership and vision of an "A" employee.

"C" employees are mediocre and don't even complete the nuts and bolts of their jobs that well. They are the hardest employees to deal with. They are not bad enough to justify dismissal, but you have to supervise them closely by holding them accountable and frequently looking over their shoulders. They don't just fail to solve problems; instead, they generate problems, leaving you to clean up the messes they create. They make poor decisions and say the wrong things to their staff members. They lack self-discipline and confidence, and are often secretly or openly disliked by the staff. They take lots of your precious time and you find yourself thinking how much easier your life would be if they weren't on your staff.

A "D" employee fails so miserably at the assigned duties that you have to dismiss them. You've made the bad mistake of picking a person for a job that they can't do. Dismissals are disruptive to your institution and morale busters. I liken firing a senior staff member to lifesaving emergency surgery. It has to be done, but it is painful and takes a long time to recover. The best policy is not to hire someone that requires you to take them to the administrative operating room.

So what is an "F" employee? If you have ever had one, you pray you won't have that experience again! An "F" employee is someone who tries to challenge your authority, polarize your staff or constituency, and take over your institution. They may try to get you thrown out. Often they have good leadership abilities, are articulate, and are deceitful. They can cause enormous trauma as they wage their war. I've inherited an "F" employee before, and the only thing good about them is that they will drive you to your knees in prayer. They have to be dealt with decisively or anarchy will result.

The more important question at this juncture is how do you find "A" employees? First of all, you have to be one yourself. This kind of staff member is more attracted than recruited. They are not put off by problems. In fact, difficult situations or problems attract them. They love the challenge. They desire good visionary leadership that is accomplishing something significant. They want a leader who will help them develop and will recognize their contribution. They want to be part of an effective team. That is why the more "A" employees you have, the easier it is to attract other "A" employees.

It is rare that a potential "A" employee walks in the door, but it occasionally happens. What you are looking for is a person with a proven record of success who has clearly demonstrated the capability of visionary leadership. The most beneficial way to assess if someone has leadership is to see who is following that person and the quality of the followers. In my experience, the best way to find "A" employees is to always be looking for them. Look for successful people who are ready to transition or are open to a change. In this regard, I'm an opportunist. Let me give you an example.

When I first arrived at CMDA, I learned that Dave, a very successful media director, was ready to transition. He had a great staff that loved and admired him, and he had previously built from scratch the best media center of any mission organization in the U.S. I was less than six months into my new job, we were getting ready to move CMDA to Bristol, and CMDA didn't even own a 35mm camera, much less have a media center. We were in debt, so we didn't even have the money to buy media equipment. But I knew that media was going to be key to our growth and development.

So I began pursuing Dave with e-mails and phone calls, and I invited him for a visit. I told him about my vision for CMDA, but was honest about the problems we faced. Dave knew me personally, and he knew my leadership style and vision. Soon, he was eager to take on the challenge and joined us in the midst of major transition and uncertainty. If you recruit "A" employees, everything else follows.

Dave, Dr. Rudd, and I built our first audio studio ourselves in the corner of a large room. I still remember offsetting the studs and building the floor on a bed of sand to dampen the noise of a nearby train track. Today, CMDA has state of the art television and audio facilities that have produced hundreds of programs and resources. Using our satellite capabilities, I have even debated cloning with an Oxford professor live on the BBC in London, England.

I could go down the list of my senior staff and tell you similar stories. Almost all of them have the capabilities to, or already have, lead their own organizations. "A" employees are like diamonds. When you find one, grab them. They take special handling to keep motivated and keep them on your staff because other organizations will try to recruit them away from you. Give them the opportunity to be part of your strategic planning. They often will pick goals even higher than you would, but more importantly, they "own" those goals. Secondly, give them the authority to make decisions and the resources to reach their goals. If you don't have the resources, give them a path and the challenge to obtain them.

As a visionary leader, that is one of the reasons I loved the system set up by World Gospel Mission, the organization I served with in Kenya. After raising your own support, you could continue to raise money for your ministry account and then transfer it to any approved budget item. It gave me a path to get the resources to start programs, build needed facilities, and even help other missionaries who were struggling to raise support. I could develop a vision and get it approved. Then I had a path to get the resources to accomplish it by raising money myself or writing a grant application.

Next, turn your "A" employees loose and give them easy access to you for feedback, affirmation, and problem solving. By easy access, I mean have an open door policy, but also schedule a regular time to meet with them on a weekly basis. They don't have to wait until their meeting for a decision or to discuss an issue. You want them to be able to keep things moving. You don't want to be their choke point. The scheduled time is used to review non-time sensitive issues, step back and look at progress towards goals, and provide encouragement and help in reaching the objectives.

Everyone has their own management styles, but the one I've found effective is based on a medical model. What do you do when you have a difficult clinical quandary? You usually grab a few key people and go to the bedside, review the patient, and make a decision on what to do next. I do the same thing in managing CMDA. If someone sticks their head in the door with a problem that involves finance and IT, I just get the key people on the phone right then or ask them to come to my office instead of waiting until a committee can meet. We take five to ten minutes for input and discussion, make a decision, and move ahead. This keeps your organization moving. It's simple. I just ask myself who needs to have input in or knowledge of what we are discussing and get them involved. I keep the train moving.

Great senior staff members are one of the keys to organizational success. Picking the right staff members will take your organization to new heights.

CHAPTER 12
MID-LEVEL MANAGERS

If you have good senior staff, the next step in creating a great team is much easier since they will select, motivate, train, equip, and supervise the next level—your supervisory staff. These are your department heads that run individual areas of your hospital or clinic. These individuals lead the medical wards, central supply, administrative departments, the lab, and other areas critical to smooth functioning.

The principles of finding the right people for these positions are similar to recruiting your senior team, but there are some important differences and additional factors you need to know.

Many mission hospitals are in remote areas, making recruitment difficult. Education for children holds high importance for trained staff, especially in countries with pyramidal educational systems. Across the nation in Kenya, students take an exam at the end of primary school, and only a small percentage of the students go on to a higher level of training. The same process is repeated at every stage of education with only the best students moving forward for additional education. It is "one strike and you're out" if you have a bad national exam day. These "school leavers" have high expectations from the education they received, yet no avenue to get a good job and support a family. Parents are very cognizant of the fact that they must get a great education for their children if they are to succeed, but often those opportunities don't exist around the mission facility.

Here is how I approached this problem as it was affecting our recruitment efforts. First, I conducted an informal assessment of our local schools. What were their strengths and weaknesses? What instructional, financial, facility, and teacher needs did they have? How was the leadership? I then developed a plan to help improve the local schools. We raised funds to get donated books shipped in for their libraries, bought supplies, and tried to help get qualified teachers involved. We had some success but still didn't get the quality we needed. A few years after I left, the hospital started its own primary school, hired great teachers, and ensured that the employees' children received an education that was at least as good or even better than anywhere else.

The hospital's greatest liability became one of its best recruiting tools. As students graduate and score well on their exams, the lure of joining your staff to get the kids into a quality school is documented and enhanced. It was worth the investment to get the kind of staff the hospital needed. Extraordinary but fundamental problems require extraordinary effort and investment.

In some locations, you face another problem in recruiting nurses, lab technicians, and other key personnel—tribalism. Those who are not from the predominate tribe around the hospital are ostracized, discriminated against, and even threatened. I was amazed when I arrived in Africa to find tribalism a greater problem than racism. Millions have died in tribal-based civil unrest in Uganda, Somalia, Sudan, and many other countries.

It is a difficult problem to deal with, but an important one to address. It is much more a spiritual than a mind issue, but it is difficult to overcome generations of bias that goes back to tribal wars of long ago. In our situation, the best measurement of the depth of an individual's walk with the Lord was the attitude towards other tribes.

It is important to deal with the problem head on with your staff. Talk about it. Preach on it. Have small group discussions about it and recruit staff from other tribes to come to your hospital. Work hard to break down the barriers. One of the best ways to do this is to have small group Bible studies in homes with a mixture of tribes involved. As individuals get to know each other more intimately and draw closer to God, they draw closer to each other.

Even if you are successful in addressing these efforts, it still may be hard to get the quality staff members you need in a remote area. They may be unwilling to come because of the lack of other amenities. Or they might be willing to come but are not trained. The answer may be to start your own training school.

When I arrived at Tenwek, we had only six trained staff in our 135-bed hospital. Everyone else had been trained on the job as ward attendants, medicine dispensers, or outpatient staff. We knew we needed to start a training school, but we had the chicken and egg problem. Our nurses had more than enough work to do in the wards and we couldn't spare them to teach. Yet without doing that, we would never adequately staff our facility. Many of them did not have the desire or abilities to be a good teacher. We were never going to improve the hospital until we started a nursing school.

I realized we needed a firm goal that everyone could work toward in order to get where we needed to go. We strategically decided that a nurse training facility was a top priority which merited our time and efforts. We looked at our strengths, weaknesses, problems, and present resources. We took the time to visit a number of missionary nursing schools to ask what was going well, where their major problems were, and what they would do differently if they started all over again. We asked ourselves, "If it was possible to do this seemingly impossible thing, what would be the first step?" We knew we would need classrooms and demonstration labs, so we designed those into our next building project. Every major project has inertia and the hardest thing is to get the ball rolling and picking up speed. When people see something happening, they want to get onboard and begin to believe that the dream is going to become a reality.

To make a long story short, it took four or five years to raise the funds, build the classrooms, recruit an experienced missionary nurse with the right degrees and vision to lead the school, deal with the nursing board, write a curriculum, and much more. We started at the lowest level of training—we enrolled community nurses and then upgraded the school to the registered nursing school level.

It was worth the effort. Over time, the nursing school became the engine to revamp, revitalize, and upgrade our hospital's quality. Within a decade or so, the school's graduates were scoring in the top ten on the national qualifying exam. More importantly, each nurse was bonded to work at the hospital for a couple of years after graduation where we mentored, observed, and then recruited the most successful to stay at the hospital on a long-term basis. We gave opportunities to our present staff to enter the school; later on, we sent the best of them on for more specialized training. We'll spend more time discussing training programs in a later chapter.

The most important insight we had was to realize that our goal was to train missionary nurses, to reproduce ourselves, and to realize that discipling students was as important as the knowledge and skills they learned. They would go out to influence other hospitals and clinics from urban to the most remote and difficult areas if we did our job well.

Developing training schools is difficult, but it ensures a steady supply of high quality staff members who are likely to want to stay in your locale. In addition to the nursing school, we started a laboratory technician school and a chaplaincy training program to meet our needs and help other mission facilities.

As an organization becomes larger, more structure is needed. It becomes harder to manage without a framework. We've already talked about the importance of job descriptions in order for your supervisory staff, as well as the people they manage, to know their purpose, duties, and responsibilities. You then need to "marry" individual standards of performance to each person's job description.

Standards of performance let employees know when they do a good job. They give you a measurement tool with which to evaluate and develop your staff. If done properly, they increase morale and help your employees feel confident in their places within the organization.

Here is how you develop these standards. Take the list of duties from the employee's job description and attach this statement to it: "I will have done this duty satisfactorily when…." Let me give you an example. A nurse in charge of a ward may have a duty "to administer medications to patients." The standard for that duty could read, "I will have administered medications to patients satisfactorily when all patients receive their medications within fifteen minutes of the scheduled time and there is less than one dispensing error per month."

Standards should be measurable and checkable. An example of an inadequate standard would be "to improve medication dispensing practices." Improve is a nebulous term that can't be verified. For example, someone involved in fundraising would set a goal to improve giving to the annual fund. That could be $1 more or $100,000 more. Of course, a huge difference exists between the two. By being specific, staff members know if they are meeting the standards set.

A duty can have more than one standard. I always aim to measure quality and quantity by answering the questions: "How well should it be done?" and "How often or to what accuracy?" Someone who has the responsibility to supervise subordinates may have standards like meet for a thirty-minute supervisory section every week, conduct an annual review with each employee, bring patient complaints to the responsible employee's attention within twenty-four hours, etc.

The skill to develop standards of performance (SOP) should be taught to each employee and they should initially draw up their own list. This gives ownership and causes them to think critically about their jobs. It gets them to set their own goals and buy into the system. The supervisor then sits down with the employee and goes over the standards to make sure they are realistic, yet challenging. SOPs should be evaluated periodically and adjusted. Some are set too low and others too high. Some are set appropriately and then accomplished and you are just ratcheting up the goal to improve performance.

SOPs should definitely be reviewed at least at the annual performance review and filed with the employee's job description. They are a great means to give staff positive feedback and set goals for continual improvement. Some standards may be deleted if found not to be important or an adequate measurement of success with others put in as replacements. They will do a lot to improve the quality of healthcare you provide. Supervisory staff should not only have them, but should also make sure each staff member they supervise has them as well.

SOPs work because of a basic principle—what gets measured gets done. It makes sense. Just talk to any student or employee. Students always want the teacher to tell them if "that will be on the test." In other words, is that going to be measured? If so, I will pay attention to it. Standards of performance tell the employee not only what to pay attention to, but allow them to self-evaluate how well they are doing.

Let's talk about annual evaluations. First of all, they should be done. Their purpose is to catch people doing something good and help them develop. I always ask staff to evaluate themselves based on their job description, standards of performance, and a self-evaluation questionnaire. I then prepare a written response to what they did and give it back to them along with a formal evaluation I filled out. We then meet to discuss them. Almost all the time, this is an opportunity for positive feedback, goal setting, and dealing with difficulties they are facing—relationally, personally, education, or tools they need to do the job.

Problems should not be put off until the performance review. You want to catch problems early and deal with them while they are small and fresh in the employee's mind and your mind. You want to do this privately, politely, and with the right attitude. Remember, God has entrusted each of your employees to your care. You have a stewardship responsibility to help meet their spiritual, professional, financial, emotional, and developmental needs. In correcting staff members, your goal is to help them to develop into all that God designed them to be. Let me give you an example.

Mary has been late for work three out of five days in the last week. She is a supervisor, so the Nursing Officer In-charge (NOIC) you've helped train asks to meet with her and says, "Thanks for coming by, Mary. Sit down; I need a few minutes of your time. I've been watching your work and want to compliment you on the way you care for patients. You show real compassion and are providing good care. There is one thing I need to bring up, though. You have been getting to work late. Do you have some problem in getting to the hospital on time that I need to be aware of?"

Note the NOIC is giving positive feedback and reaffirming the good things the employee is doing. She is polite, but clearly identifies the problem. She asks an open-ended question to find out if there are other things going on before jumping to a judgment like "you are too lazy to get out of bed on time." Mary's watch may have broken and she hasn't had time to replace it. She may have a sick child, transportation problems, or many other things affecting her arrival time. The NOIC may have suggestions or resources to help her solve her problem. It also gives Mary an opportunity to shoulder the blame for the problem and address it herself.

After Mary responds, the NOIC needs to deal with the issue. If Mary is irresponsible, the NOIC needs to tell her that. The standard expected needs to be reiterated. If the problem continues, Mary needs to be told the consequences that will follow. The NOIC needs to make sure those consequences are fair and enforced.

Each disciplinary session should be recorded in writing and put in the employee's file. If the person does not respond, they may then need to be on probation for a short period, given a written expectation, and told that this is the last chance.

Here is how I terminate an employee. I say, "John, I made a mistake. I hired you for a job you couldn't do. Your failure in performing your duties is as much my problem as it is yours. I've put a lot of effort in trying to train and supervise you to see if we can get this solved, but we haven't made adequate progress. Unfortunately, I'm going to have to let you go." I then try to show love and concern for them with a small severance package of two weeks' salary or whatever is appropriate. When you fire someone, immediately move that person out of your institution and have someone else pick up the vacated duties. Leaving a terminated employee to grouse and complain will poison your staff relationships as they try to recruit others to their side.

There are many aspects involved in running a good healthcare service, but doing it well ensures patients get the care they need and creates a working atmosphere that glorifies the Lord.

CHAPTER 13
STRATEGIC PLANNING

Yogi Bera, the baseball diamond philosopher, said, "If you don't know where you are going, you might end up somewhere else." Long before Yogi Bera quipped, doctor Luke wrote, "Suppose one of you wants to build a tower. Will he not first sit down and estimate the cost to see if he has enough money to complete it?" (Luke 14:28, NIV 1984). Strategic planning is a key to success in most endeavors, and this includes missionary medicine.

With all the patients waiting to be seen, surgeries to perform, and prayer letters to write, why bother planning? Because entropy happens. Without goals and a clear mission, your outreach becomes disorganized, inefficient, and unresponsive to the changes continuously occurring around you. Less important details easily obscure the path to real progress. You are distracted by the noise of the urgent and don't put your effort into the strategic activities that will have the greatest long-term impact. Money and personnel are directed to nonproductive activities. How do I know? I've been there—overwhelmed and directionless in the face of seemingly insurmountable problems. Without a clear vision and strategies, staff members at all levels lose hope in the future.

When I arrived at CMDA in 1994, the organization had just completed a three-month campaign to wipe out the year's large projected deficit. Unfortunately, nothing causing the deficit was changed. The organization had been without an executive director for almost a year, the mission arm was threatening to break off and become its own organization, and my newly inherited staff was disillusioned and discouraged. That was just the tip of the iceberg of the problems I uncovered in the first few months.

How did I start to turn things around? I spent a few months learning everything I could about the staff, board, programs, and needs of Christian doctors. I then sat down and wrote a strategic plan. It was a "quick and dirty" plan, but it had measurable goals and clear strategies. It was comprehensive as it addressed every aspect of the organization and looked five years into the future. I then took it to the board for approval. The board had never seen a CMDA strategic plan and had fallen into the trap of micromanaging the organization. They were thrilled to see a road map to success and, with some training, turned their attention to measuring progress toward our agreed upon goals instead of trying to run the organization during three meetings a year. The CMDA staff was excited to clearly see the journey ahead and to mark each milestone we passed. We made more progress in those five years than any in recent memory because we had a plan.

Before we finished those five years, I was determined to make the next five-year plan even better. We budgeted and brought in an outside professional facilitator to consult with us. We formed a strategic planning committee made up of the top administrators and a select group of the board and took them through a nine-month planning process. It involved a survey of our members to assess their needs and four weekend meetings completely focused on planning for the future. A board has the responsibility to set goals for the organization, and strategic planning is the way to enable its members to do their job.

Thinking back I can draw an analogy to barn building. The first time, I saw we desperately needed a barn, so I built one quickly by myself. We had never had a barn, so everyone was pleased, even though the barn was far from perfect. The second barn was better because I involved others in its planning. This time, I wanted to get everyone who used the barn involved in the planning. Because the barn was much bigger and more complicated, they knew what they needed to do in their areas of the barn, and by helping to design the barn they "owned" it. This time, I got the heads of all CMDA's departments to help construct the strategic plan along with the board. Our senior staff had two separate days off-site devoted to strategic planning, and then we took our ideas to the strategic planning committee set up by the board. We had done so much work that the board polished it up in a day and a half. We now have the best strategic plan we have ever had.

I'm convinced that strategic planning is the tool to help you create the future the way it ought to be. It will help you and others measure organizational progress and personal performance. So how do you do it if you have never constructed a strategic plan? Let me take you through the process step by step.

First, commit yourself to doing it. It is going to take some of your valuable time, but it will be worth the investment.

Secondly, get others from your leadership team and your board involved. If your board doesn't see the importance of having a small group of its members go through the process with you, do it just with your staff the first time and then take it to the board for approval. Your planning team can be six to ten people, but there is no hard and fast number. It should be big enough to bring in all perspectives and sufficient ideas but small enough to function well and not get bogged down. If board members are involved, they should make up about half the team. The full board ultimately approves the plan the committee puts together.

Plans fail for lack of counsel, but with many advisers they succeed (Proverbs 15:22, NIV 1984).

Thirdly, get the planning team committed to prayer before and during the process. You want the Lord's direction and guidance. You want to know His plan for the future of your ministry.

There is no wisdom, no insight, no plan that can succeed against the Lord (Proverbs 21:30, NIV 1984).

Commit to the Lord whatever you do, and your plans will succeed (Proverbs 16:3, NIV 1984).

If possible, get away from your institution to eliminate interruptions and distractions. You don't have to go far or to an expensive site. If it is impossible to get away, have everyone clear their schedules as best they can. You can accomplish a great deal in a well-planned day, but realize that the process may take multiple days to do it right depending on the complexity of your institution and the number of its programs.

Make the planning fun. Take breaks, use humor, and have food available. Use a video projector/computer, a blackboard, pens, and a white board to have each section of the plan available for everyone to see and edit. Make sure you have an easy way to erase and improve suggestions. I've found it helpful to separate brainstorming from critiquing times. Though critiquing is necessary, it can stifle creativity when you mix the two. Someone should facilitate the process and make sure everyone is involved. If you can find an experienced outside facilitator, that is ideal; if not, go ahead with who you have available.

One very helpful detail during the process is to identify your "stakeholders." Who has a stake in your ministry? Patients? The church? Community leaders? Missions? Staff members? Staff families? Answering this question is a great place to start.

For CMDA, the list contains our members, our member representatives, our board, and our staff. For your hospital, it might be the people in your catchment area, your governing body, your staff, your church, and even your government if it has some sort of control over your ministry. Stakeholders are those who value the success of your ministry. You want to keep them informed, involved, and content with the job you are doing. If you don't keep them happy, you will have problems that could affect the very future of your ministry.

Secondly, list the beneficiaries of your organization's services. For CMDA, it includes medical, dental, physician assistant, and podiatry students as well as graduates, their spouses, the church, the government, and our culture. For you, it might be the church, your mission, your patient population, and the Ministry of Health if you are in an institution. Knowing your beneficiaries helps you realize what goals, objectives, and strategies you should design to serve them. It also tells you what you should not be doing.

Recently, one of our members wanted me to help start an organization to bring conservative Jewish, Protestant, and Catholic bioethicists together for networking, writing, and conferences to impact the bioethics agenda in our country. This is a good project that could impact our culture, but I quickly realized that conservative bioethicists are not part of our target group of beneficiaries. Doing this would distract us from who we are here to serve.

After you've identified them, survey or interview the key stakeholders. What are you doing well? What are you doing poorly? What do they desire from your ministry? Where would they like the ministry to be in five years? Get specific and make sure to get adequate information from all stakeholders.

This data is invaluable to helping in the planning, so you want to spend time with your team figuring out what is important for you to know from your survey as you plan.

When we did our survey, we learned, unbeknownst to us, that 75 percent of CMDA members had been involved in domestic or overseas missions in the last two years. We thought the percentage would be much lower than that. Most of them had done those activities with other groups. So we began to ask ourselves, "What about our short-term mission experiences should be different to make them the best? What was the most important thing that should happen on a trip—evangelism, medical care, church growth, or participant transformation?" We agreed that participant transformation would have the greatest long-term impact so it should be of highest importance. We then developed strategies to make it happen and decided how to measure success in that area so we would know we had accomplished our goal.

As you collect survey data, don't forget to analyze the information you already have. Look at your ministry for the last five years. What are the trends in admissions and out-patient visits? Are disease patterns changing? Are your patients coming from greater distances? What happened through your spiritual ministry? Is it growing deeper and wider? Where is your bed occupancy heading? Is your lab able to handle its load? Graph out important data to do a better trend analysis. Various members of your team can collect portions of the data and present it at the next team meeting.

After collecting and analyzing the information you need, meet with your team to do a S.W.O.T. analysis by answering these questions:

1. What are your **strengths**?
2. What are your **weaknesses**?
3. What are your strategic **opportunities**?
4. What are the **threats** to your ministry?

Among your strengths may be a good reputation in the community, stable leadership, good government relations, and more. You may be weak financially, not have adequate trained national staff, or lack career missionary personnel. You may see an opportunity to open a training school, expand your dispensary system, or increase the number of beds to meet your demand. Your ministry may be threatened by poor economics, government instability, or increasing import restrictions. Clearly identifying each of these areas gives you a clearer picture of where you are and suggests how you should move forward. Write them down and put this data along with the other information you have collected in a notebook for each of your team members.

Now you start putting together the components of your strategic plan by writing your:

1. Mission
2. Vision
3. Core Values
4. Key Result Areas
5. Goals
6. Objectives
7. Strategies

Mission
"If you don't know where you're going, it doesn't matter which way you go." - Cheshire cat in Lewis Carroll's *Alice in Wonderland*

It's ironic that many mission medical facilities do not have a clearly articulated mission statement. Yet, it is the key to knowing where you are going and how to get there. It is the yardstick you hold next to everything you do. If you don't have a mission statement, put one together at your next board meeting. If you have one, it is time to review it.

The best mission statement is a one-sentence, clear, concise statement that says what the organization is, what it does, who it serves, and to what end. Some statements also set geographical boundaries. "CMDA exists to motivate, train, and equip Christian physicians and dentists to glorify God." That is short and easily memorized, because everyone in your organization should know and be able to share the mission of the organization with others.

It is important to clearly state your goal in the mission statement and not just the method. Your goal is not to treat the sick. That is a method. Your goal might be to "make people healthy in body, mind, and spirit." Sometimes people want more detail to guide the organization's growth and functions. CMDA does this by saying,

"The Christian Medical & Dental Associations exists to motivate, educate, and equip Christian physicians and dentists to glorify God by:

- living out the character of Christ in their homes, practices, communities, and around the world;
- pursuing professional competence and Christ-like compassion in their daily work;
- influencing their families, colleagues, and patients toward a right relationship with Jesus Christ;
- advancing biblical principles in bioethics and health to the church and society."

The short sentence is what everyone knows to share with others. The longer version guides the board and administration in evaluating present and potential programs to see if they accomplish our mission. It shares more about methods and intermediary ends. Note that the first sentence is the core mission statement which is memorable and succinct. The sub-points describe our playing field and put fences around it. CMDA has more than 40 different outreaches. So our playing field is large, but it still has boundaries which are further defined by the board policy manual. All the same, everything we do fits within this mission statement.

A mission hospital in Africa might have a mission statement like, "The mission of Hope Hospital's healthcare system is to bring health and hope in Christ to the people of north central Zambia."

Note that this mission statement sets geographical boundaries. If this group started work in the south of the country, it would be working outside its mission statement. "Bring health" could encompass curative and preventive programs, training programs, and even economic development that improves health.

Vision
A vision statement encapsulates what it will look like when you are accomplishing your mission. They are often catchy slogans. At Tenwek Hospital, "We treat, Jesus heals" is emblazoned on the entrance sign as the hospital's vision statement. The National Forest Service vision statement states it is "caring for the land and serving the people."

Where there is no vision, the people perish (Proverbs 29:18a, KJV).

Develop a vision statement by answering the question, "I see...." Make the vision statement pithy and memorable.

In 1994, CMDA's vision and slogan was, "A Fellowship of Christian Doctors." Not too awe inspiring! I pointed out to the board that fellowship was not a vision but a by-product of working together toward a common goal. We changed our vision statement to "Changing Hearts in Healthcare." It was better, but later we went a step further with a revised vision, "Transformed Doctors, Transforming the World."

Our vision was not only to transform the hearts and minds of our members, but to see them changing the hearts and minds of others as they witnessed and served.

Good mission and vision statements are hard to develop. I find it is good to work hard, let it gel, and then come back to it again. Then bounce it off others to get their reaction and input and work some more until you get something that everyone can grab onto. Once you have it, put it out to everyone you can in every way you can. Combine it with a good logo and it will be your trademark.

Core Values
Your next task in strategic planning is to develop your values statement. Your values statement displays your guiding principles on how your organization will act as you carry out the strategic plan. In one

sense, they are the rules governing your organization and the standards defining your character and reputation. They are targeted to your staff and board to set ethical, knowledge, and behavioral standards, and to the public to reassure them that you can be trusted. It is your covenant with your employees on what you consider to be the most important values that they must live out. That is why, along with your mission and vision, values are posted around the workplace to remind everyone of the standards expected.

CMDA has eight core values. We covenant to be:

- Christ-like
- Controlled by the Holy Spirit
- Committed to Scripture
- Communing in Prayer
- Compassionate
- Competent
- Courageous
- Culturally Relevant

We use Scripture to legitimize each of our values. We sum them up with our staff at the end of each chapel service by challenging them to "go and be godly."

Note that half of CMDA's values focus on our spiritual relationship with God and the other four describe how we will relate to our constituency. Of course, there are many values you might want to consider. Pick those most important for your ministry. A total of eight is actually more than I would suggest and they don't have to all begin with the same letter! I would think Christ-like, competent, and compassionate would be on any healthcare outreach list. You may want to add evangelistic and holistic to your list and go with five values. The key is to agree on your key values with your leaders and then ruthlessly promote them in word, writing, and action to your staff.

The mission, vision, and core values should be formally reviewed at least every five years, more often if your board or administration has a major turnover. Everyone needs to discuss the nuances of your core documents and invest in them. These statements need to be posted in your institution as a reminder to you, your staff, and patients.

Key Result Areas

What are the key indicators showing you are accomplishing your mission? Key Result Areas are broad descriptions under which all of your goals, objectives, and strategies dwell. These areas should be limited to no more than four to six areas so you and everyone else can easily remember them.

These areas help organize all the things your ministry does in order to help you and your staff further describe how you carry out your mission. They also are an important way to communicate with your constituency, funders, church, and government organizations. In other words you say, "Our mission is…and our key result areas are what we do to accomplish and complete our mission."

Here is an example. To accomplish CMDA's mission, we focus on five Key Result Areas:

1. <u>Transformation</u> – Ministries that transform medical professionals' lives through evangelism and discipleship.
2. <u>Service</u> – Ministries that provide opportunities for doctors and others to use their God-given skills to meet the needs of others and share the gospel with them.
3. <u>Equipping</u> – Resources and services that give medical professionals and the church the knowledge and tools they need to effectively serve the Lord.
4. <u>Voice</u> – Outreaches that speak for our members to the government, media, church, and public on bioethical and public policy issues while also training Christians to be effective advocates themselves.
5. <u>Organizational Capacity</u> – The personnel, structure, and resources to accomplish our mission.

All of our ministries fit under these Key Result Areas, and each individual ministry has its own goals, objectives, and strategies.

Let's look at Key Result Areas (KRAs) as they could be articulated if you were working in a mission hospital.

1. Curative – Under this, you might put your health centers, dispensaries, outpatient department, surgical department, etc.

2. Preventive – Under this area, you would put your community health and community development work. You might also add your inpatient health education department.
3. Training – This KRA would have your nursing school, your laboratory technologist school, and your family practice residency program.
4. Evangelism and Discipleship – This KRA could include your chaplaincy department, your new convert follow-up program, your staff discipleship program, etc.
5. Organizational Capacity – This area would include your information technology, finance, housekeeping, security, maintenance, and other similar departments.

To monitor your work as you strive to complete your mission, you would examine how well you are doing in each of these specific areas.

Goals, Objectives, and Strategies
We are now down to the nuts and bolts of your strategic plan—goals, objectives, and strategies. Goals are the changes you want to achieve. They tend to be broad and are sometimes harder to quantify than objectives.

CMDA's first goal is to "Transform doctors into the character of Christ and to influence their colleagues and patients toward a right relationship with Jesus Christ." That is a big concept just below the level of our Key Result Area of "Transformation." It is difficult to measure transformed doctors, but it can be done! Goals are a phrase or a succinct sentence in length.

A healthcare ministry might have a goal to "prevent disease among our target population." Below each goal, it is wise to add a short paragraph titled "Rationale" that explains why working towards this goal will accomplish your mission. This rationale helps keep you on track.

If your organization is large, you may want to break down your main goal into sub-goals to accomplish it. We took our first goal and created sub-goals for the Campus & Community Ministries outreach, the Side By Side ministry for doctor's spouses, and other areas. You may want to have sub-goals for preventing disease in your community health work, your outpatient department, your HIV outreach, and your clinic system.

Under Campus & Community Ministries, our first sub-goal is to "train graduate leadership and develop chapters and councils." We follow that with the strategy of redirecting our regional and area directors toward a major effort in establishing and equipping key graduate doctor leaders for local communities and student groups.

Our measurable objectives follow. Objectives must be quantifiable and have a deadline. They hold the overall leader accountable to your governing body and each part of your ministry accountable to the leader of it. They tell you clearly whether you are succeeding or not and what area needs more attention. To be effective, these must be reviewed regularly. Objectives serve another purpose in that they can give your senior staff satisfaction. Completed objectives let staff members know they are doing their jobs well and that they will be recognized for it.

So here is the first section of our strategic plan. It contains the first nine of our 250 individual measurable objectives.

1. TRANSFORMATION
   - Goal - To transform doctors into the character of Christ and to influence their colleagues and patients toward a right relationship with Jesus Christ.
   - Rationale - CMDA exists to help doctors and other healthcare professionals grow into all that God designed them to be. Through evangelizing and discipling during the training and graduate years, CMDA desires to bring doctors to Christ and help them become like the Great Physician. This involves continually deepening their relationship with the Savior and learning how to apply biblical principles to every aspect of life.
   - Campus & Community Ministries
     1. Train graduate leadership and develop more chapters/councils.
        i. Strategy - Redirect the regional and area directors toward a major effort in establishing and equipping key graduate doctor leaders for local communities and student groups.

ii. Objectives
- Two graduate leaders for every city over 150,000 by <date>
- Four graduate leaders for every medical/dental school (one for each class) by <date>
- Develop and maintain a database of existing local councils and chapters with leaders and their contact information identified in <date>
- Set up monthly national communication with leaders in <date>
- Have 80 councils by <date>
- Fund and hire a dental director for a two-year trial in <year>
- Yearly campus advisor and council conference by <year>
- Integrate graduate ministry with local churches at ten sites where CMDA works through a local church in ministry by <year>
- Develop small group model of local ministry in twenty cities that have ongoing small group discussion (four couples) centered around JAWs by <year>

A strategic plan is a dynamic document at the lowest levels, but less so as you move up through it. You may accomplish an objective much earlier than anticipated, find it is more difficult than you imagined, or even determine after you start that it is not worth doing. We change a few objectives every four months when we systematically review our plan.

So if your goal is to prevent disease in your target population, it might look like this.

1. PREVENT DISEASE
   - Goal - To prevent disease among our catchment's population.
   - Rationale - Our mission is to improve the health of our target population. Through our curative services we attempt to cure, but we will better reduce suffering and prevent death through a vigorous effort to teach better health-related behavior and by targeting specific interventions to prevent serious illness.

- Community Health
    1. Motivate, train, and equip two hundred Community Health Workers by March <year>
        i. Strategy - Mobilize the community to understand their health issues, set up Community Health Committees, and have them help select, supervise, and motivate health volunteers we train in the community.
        ii. Objectives
            - Apply for grant funding by November <year>
            - Pick thirty target village groups by the end of <year>
            - Conduct a baseline survey of ten leading health indicators by March <year>
            - Select, train, and supervise ten Community Health Committees a year for the next three years
            - Develop a health and evangelistic curriculum by March <year>
            - Hold four-week CHW training sessions with three to four groups every four months starting in April <year>
            - Hire three Community Health Supervisors by April <year> and add two more in year three
            - Do a follow-up survey to measure impact in January <year>

The goal would be even better if you had a baseline survey of health indicators and a target number for each to attach to or you could include these as sub-goals to the main goal.

Goals, strategies, and objectives take time to develop but are like a road map. Would you say, "I'm going to visit a remote village in Nepal," and then just walk out the door? Of course not. You would plan your modes of transport, make sure the time schedule worked, identify what you need for the trip, and prepare a budget estimate. If you did that, you would get there most of the time. A strategic plan tells you where you want to go, how you are going to get there, how much it is going to cost in money and time, and when you will arrive. The first time you conduct a strategic planning meeting, it is helpful to have an outside facilitator. This experienced person takes you through the process step by step. This facilitator doesn't determine the content, but explains what you need to accomplish in each part of your plan and ensures that you accomplish it well.

Take time to plan. I know you are busy, but this is worth your time. Your foundational documents put your ministry and institution on the road to success; they bind your staff, church leaders, and board into a common purpose; they guide your development; and they "brand" your outreach to those you serve.

PART 4
ORGANIZATIONAL MONITORING

CHAPTER 14
DEVELOPING THE CHRISTIAN WORKPLACE

What an unexpected surprise and honor! *Christianity Today* and the Christian Management Association gave CMDA the first "Best Christian Workplace in the U.S." award several years ago after surveying and interviewing our staff. As you can imagine, other organizations contacted us asking for the secret of our success. I confess I had to sit down and put into words some of the principles guiding us. Some were so ingrained that we had not even thought about them.

I want to share those with you but also take it a little further by walking down memory lane. How would I apply these principles in a medical missions outreach if I were back in missions and doing what you are doing today? Though the applications may be different, the principles are the same whether you are running a large mission hospital, managing a clinic, in charge of a community health program, or running CMDA.

Do not misunderstand me. CMDA is not the perfect workplace. We have our problems. Like you, I have had to fire people, solve interpersonal conflicts, calm irate constituents, deal with financial shortfalls, revamp governance structures, and much more. However, when followed, what principals are most likely to create a workplace where staff members are joyous, fulfilled, and working hard for the Lord?

Rally Around the Mission
You have to know where you are going before people will rally to the cause. Corporately, that means developing clear purpose, mission, vision, values, and goal documents. With staff, it is answering the questions, "Why should I invest my life in this?" and "Will it make a

difference for the kingdom?" You want everyone involved to see the organization's mission as their mission and feel it is so important that they are eager to get up every morning to do it. This is done on many levels but let me give you an example.

We just talked about CMDA's old slogan, "A Fellowship of Christian Doctors." Does that stir your heart? Are you willing to shout that as your battle cry? No, of course not. Fellowship is important, but it is the by-product of being in mission together. We changed our slogan to "Changing the Face of Healthcare, By Changing the Hearts of Doctors," which later morphed into "Changing Hearts in Healthcare."

We rally around our mission in publications to our members, but we also rally around it with our staff. We share stories of how the mission is being accomplished. We dream up new ways to accomplish it. I talk about our mission every chance I get. Employees need to know that what they are doing is important and that they are making a difference.

Adopt Instead of Hiring
As we discussed earlier, we do not hire senior staff; instead, we adopt them into our family. We will not settle for a potential "C" employee, but look for only "A" ones. If you do that, there will be an exponential multiplication effect in impact. That is why Dr. Rudd and I are always involved in hiring key people. Of course, we look for people with the right skills but they also must be called by God to work at CMDA. If we do not sense that, we do not hire them. They also must have the personality, work ethic, and spiritual depth to complement and enhance our staff mix. One bad apple can spoil the whole bushel.

Does that mean everyone is the same? No. That would be like making breakfast bread with only flour but no yeast, shortening, raisins, or cinnamon. Your workplace ingredients must blend so that the sum is more than the parts. Hiring staff is serious business and is one of the most important things leaders do. For lower level staff, we utilize our best staff at the level above them to make the decision.

The other aspect of adoption versus hiring is that I contract for services for a certain amount of work when hiring. In adoption, I take on a stewardship responsibility to nurture, train, cherish, encourage, discipline, and develop the individual God entrusted to my sphere of influence.

Create a Caring Atmosphere
More than ever, people need community. This is more true in the United States—where community is breaking down—than in many other countries, but we have a basic human need to be loved and cared about by others. It is impossible to carry out our stewardship responsibility unless we are involved in individual lives. That goes beyond making sure they are doing their job to cultivating genuine relationships bearing the fruits of kindness. Actions are much more important than words. Dr. Rudd is much better at this than I am, since I am on the road so much. He calls to meet needs when employees are sick, goes and sits in the emergency room, visits in the hospital, or gives medical advice. He helps people move, does counseling, and many other caring things. He creates an atmosphere and sets a standard that others emulate.

Staff members at CMDA genuinely care about each other and express it in concrete ways. Each year at our staff Christmas party, we have an ornament exchange. Whoever's ornament you get becomes your prayer partner for the year. Many staff do special things for their prayer partner throughout the year.

One of the barriers to a caring community is the "great divide" that can exist between missionary and national staff. There may be a caring atmosphere among the missionaries but little going on across the deep valley. Address this in practical ways. Invite key staff over for meals, start a Bible study in your home, work on something together outside the medical/dental work situation, visit their homes, offer to help them with a personal project, or love on their children. In medicine, patients first want to know that you care. It is the same in the workplace.

Grow in Christ Together
At Tenwek, we used to have chapel for patients in various places simultaneously in the hospital every day. If I were to do it over, I would have chapel service for my staff during work hours at different times twice a week so everyone could attend. Employees who worship together are drawn together as they grow closer to Christ. These should

be high quality services with a variety of speakers from inside and outside the workplace. We have chapel twice a week at CMDA. We bring in special speakers, use PowerPoint, watch music videos, and learn through training courses. We never want chapel to get stale and each service must meet attendees at their point of need.

One of our former staff members was a very successful pastor who served as the staff chaplain and organized, led, and evaluated our spiritual ministry. He was also available for counseling and encouragement. The deepest bonds are forged in the fire of seeing Christ working in our lives and our co-workers' lives.

Timeliness
We get so busy working that we fail to deal with problems and issues in a timely manner. We need to have our antennas up to snoop out interpersonal frictions, overworked staff, and underperforming employees. We need to identify what isn't working and could be tuned up, and what isn't working and is beyond salvage. Most importantly, we need to deal with problems quickly.

I like to garden but hate to pull weeds. If I do not do it frequently, the small, easy-to-remove weeds turn into deeply invasive, almost immovable parasites that damage the growth of fruit and disrupt the root systems of other plants when removed.

The same is true in the workplace. The postponement of dealing with problems, especially people problems, always makes the situation worst. It also damages morale and destroys trust in leadership. Deal with issues when they are small in a loving but uncompromising manner. As with your children, staff members need to know where their boundaries are and what happens when they are crossed. We set up a system of verbal cautions, written warnings, and probation tools to use in dealing with underperforming or problem people. We work hard to salvage every one of our adoptees due to our stewardship responsibility, but staff members see that we do not shy away from hard decisions or ignore difficult problems.

Labor laws and cultural mores impact how you can deal with employee situations in many countries. You may have to adapt your techniques to the local situation, but it is critical that you deal with little problems before they become big ones. You must also do so in a consistent and Christ-like manner. That is the key to building confidence in you as a leader.

Transparency
Make sure you and other leaders are clearly seen for who you are, for the decisions being made, and for where the organization is heading. Transparency means employees can see both the good and the bad. On a personal level, share your own spiritual struggles and the ways God is teaching and maturing you. Don't hide your life behind a mirage of being a super-saint. Recently, I listened to a riveting message on forgiveness by Chuck Swindoll. It was so compelling and unforgettable because his wife Cynthia shared about conflicts with and alienation from her extended family, her own depression, and suicidal ideation. Her transparency ministered to me.

In a cross-cultural situation, this has to be done in the right manner, but it is still important. It lets others see that you are not perfect and God continues to work in you. Apologize when you wrong someone, admit your bad decisions, and confess your mistakes.

Be transparent at an organizational level as well. To feel a sense of ownership of the ministry, staff members need to know what is going on. At the same time, teach them what needs to be kept in the workplace family and what they may tell others. Ask them to pray for you and other leaders within the organization and be open to their care and counsel.

Make Memories Frequently
Look for any excuse to have fun together. We work hard and play hard at CMDA. One time, we sensed everyone had spring fever on a beautiful day, so we had a surprise "Banana Split Party" with ice cream and all the toppings. I then announced that I thought "split" should mean that we all leave work early by a couple of hours! It is surprising how fast people can shut down their computers and get into their cars!

We involve our staff in planning our parties and I'm always willing and ready to be the one laughed at. At our Christmas get-together one year, we played "Celebrity Hollywood Squares." They gave nine staff members a bag with a costume in it that they had to put on. I was

Elvis. It was a whole other me with a white sequined jumpsuit, cape, and fake sideburns! We always have a staff member photograph the craziness and put it up on the staff-only part of our website. (No, I'm not going to give you the URL!) The employees rush home to show their families all the fun we had and regularly visit the site with other employees for a few more belly laughs. We also have events for everyone to bring their spouses and children three times each year.

When Dr. Rudd and I turned fifty years old within a few months of each other, the staff picked us up out of our offices in wheelchairs for a "Fifties Party." Everyone dressed the part and my assistant brought in sundaes on roller skates. The cakes looked like vinyl records and I ended up getting a pie in the eye before the event was over.

One spring, we celebrated Easter by hiding more than one hundred plastic eggs full of goodies and one grand prize throughout the offices. It took more than two weeks for them all to be found. We regularly put together competitions, contests, and other activities to make memories and lots of conversation.

I guess you get the picture. Shared memories bind us together. In the midst of a busy work schedule in a medical mission situation, you need emotional release. Laughter is great medicine so organize a game night, put together a fun contest, or have a party. People will work better for it.

Don't Get Stuck in a Rut
Traditions are important, but variety is the spice of life. Take this situation, for example. I've been on a thousand or more forgettable airplane trips, but I still remember getting on a late night Southwest flight from San Antonio to Dallas because the stewardesses had dressed for bed with housecoats, curlers, and the yucky green face mask that some women put on for their complexion. They told us that they were trying to get us guys ready for what we were going to see when we got home! It was hilarious and unpredictable.

At CMDA, I continually emphasize that there is a better way to do everything and all of us should be out to find it. I've also been known to say, "If you don't like change, don't work here!" Like high performance race cars, a high performance organization must be continually tuned. The key is to get everyone working on the car together. Everyone's ideas are equal so we have a suggestion box and an open door policy to our offices. We take every opportunity available to brag on an individual's good idea.

We also keep barriers between departments low by encouraging staff to help each other out whenever we can. I recently had a weekly meeting with one of my department heads. She had a large mailing to get out. I suggested we rent a DVD and show it on the big screen in our assembly hall and invite staff to come in with their kids and have an envelope stuffing party. This was a first for us, and it helped get us out of a rut while also creating a few memories.

Keep it Flat
As organizations grow, they can get multilayered. Some of this is mandatory or leaders can't manage well. If you are responsible for too many people, you can't meet with them regularly to motivate, guide, and supervise them. The more layers there are, the more communications and relationships become compartmentalized. Feelings of "them versus us" fester and tensions quickly escalate.

Ideally, one person can directly supervise five to ten people well. Keep your organization as "flat" as possible to avoid problems. To do this at CMDA, Dr. Rudd and I divide up senior staff and he supervises half while I supervise the other half. We meet individually with each person we supervise each week for a scheduled meeting and our doors are open if needs arise. If I'm traveling, he has full authority to make decisions. We laughingly say that we don't always make the same decisions, but we don't make any higher percentage of wrong ones! We communicate regularly and make sure that employees don't play one of us against the other.

We also manage CMDA like we care for patients. If a decision is needed, we pull together the people needed for input and make the decision then. We avoid committees that stagnate, taking decisions to the lowest common denominator. We empower staff with the authority they need to operate well and let them know what things we need to be informed of or require approval for. This system builds trust.

We work hard to build relationships with staff members who are more than one layer below us. For example, the cleaning staff comes by every day to pick up my trash. We talk about our dogs, building a house, the weather, and killing E. coli in well water, all in just a few minutes of conversation. It is important to be approachable and available.

Communicate Consistently
Communication is the oil that makes an organization work smoothly. Without it, the machinery soon seizes up. There should be "standing communications" in the form of policy manuals and other written regulations and guidelines. There should be frequent formal communication such as newsletters, staff meetings, e-mail, or bulletins, and there should be informal communication happening in and between organizational layers. Answer the standard questions of who, what, when, where, and, more importantly, why.

I heard it said of Martin Luther that he prayed at least an hour each day, but he prayed two hours if he was going to be really busy. That is not only a good spiritual principle, but also a tenet that should guide the communication within our organization. The busier things are, the more we need to go out of our way to keep people informed.

One of the most important things to communicate is the success of your product. Share stories of how your outreach is impacting lives and the words of appreciation from those you are affecting. Staff members need to be reminded at every opportunity that they are making a difference in things they deeply care about. I encourage you to examine your workplace and see which principles you do or could employ. Figure out applications that will work where you are. We can all have a best Christian workplace!

CHAPTER 15
SITUATIONAL ANALYSIS

We were sitting around the table on a Sunday afternoon in the team house in Mogadishu, Somalia. It was our custom to hold a morning service and invite some of the U.S. military personnel working with us to join us. Many were not born again, but were just cultural Christians. Still, they flocked to that service for two reasons. One was to get some good home cooking at the meal that followed the service; the second was that there were often a number of single girls on our team about the same ages as these young fellows. At lunch, there was lots of the chatter and laughter that we all longed for. It was a little normalcy in the midst of a city torn apart by a violent civil war. For a while, we could actually forget what was going on outside.

As a few people got up to help clear the table, I was in a deep discussion with a soldier who had joined us a number of times. He was a little shaken up as his platoon was ambushed the day before and one of his buddies was wounded. I could tell he needed encouragement and support. He needed someone to listen to his story, someone who also shouldered the burden of leadership in a dangerous situation.

When he told me about the ambush, I asked, "What do you do when something like that happens?" He leaned closer and said, "It depends on the situation. They like to flank you shooting from all sides, so the first thing is to understand where they are coming from, and then you know how to respond."

This is good advice for a soldier, as well as a medical missionary, but it is advice that we are often too busy to follow. We find ourselves "shooting" at the next patient's problem and failing to understand the big picture. It is not surprising that we feel like we are overrun much of the time. In your clinic, hospital, community health program, academic position, or whatever you do, this type of analysis is critical in order to understand trends, opportunities, and problems. It tells you what you need to do to avoid casualties.

This has been on my mind because I recently completed a presentation for CMDA's board on our next five-year strategic plan. In preparation, we took the time to do a situational analysis. It was an analysis we needed to do before we could decide what to do next.

Data is available on an ongoing basis for a medical missionary to collect and periodically evaluate. One of the most valuable things we started to do at Tenwek was prepare an annual report. Completed on an annual basis, this helped us to collect all our data and organize it into a written report. The process and results were extremely valuable as we looked at our bed occupancy rate, admissions, labs done, deliveries, death rates, and much more. We would look at staff patient ratios, the disease numbers we were seeing, and our financial collection rates. We took the most critical data and put it into a five-year table which clearly showed us trends in each area. That helped us identify problems, set development priorities, buy equipment, and know what missionary and national staff we needed. Disease patterns helped focus our community health work and monitor our success. For example, we saw that our new immunization strategy in the community was making a difference when our annual admissions for measles complications dropped from 427 to 23 during a five-year period.

Along with other hospital data, this annual report gave us powerful information to motivate donors to contribute to the hospital. They were thrilled to have hard data showing that we were making a real difference in health. An increase in major surgeries told us that we needed to raise funds for more operating rooms a year or two before we desperately needed them. The number of multiple and premature births demonstrated we needed to train more nurses to staff the intensive care nursery.

It's important to note that completing a situational analysis is more than just studying statistical data. You need to collect qualitative information as well. How do staff members feel about their work conditions, salary, and housing? How satisfied are your patients and would they recommend your health outreach to others?

In addition to reviewing the internal aspects of your work, don't forget to look externally as well. We were already doing a large survey of two thousand homes every two to three years for our community health work, so we started including a few questions to assess the public's view of the hospital and better understand the needs. This can also be done with focus groups of community leaders. It is best to have someone the local people will be frank with to lead these groups.

Don't forget to analyze other missionaries' opinions and concerns. It is easy to believe you know what they are thinking, but an anonymous survey can reveal many helpful comments.

We also completed an analysis with our board and senior staff members. One of our situational analysis efforts showed that church leaders were eager to have formal leadership training that we were happy to provide. Without the analysis, we would have missed this opportunity.

Sometimes it is advantageous to go further out into the field of your constituency to seek input. What does the Ministry of Health know and think about your ministry? How do the police and local public officials see your ministry? Here are some principles that can help you complete a beneficial situational analysis.

1. Put it on your "to do" list with a due date. This won't happen by chance. Repeat the process periodically.
2. Decide who has the aptitude and the discipline to lead the process.
3. Start modestly. As systems are set in place, you can add to them. Get the most important information first.
4. Put the results in writing in a report that you can share with other leaders—your senior staff, board, church leaders, funding organization, mission executives, etc.
5. Take the information from your situational analysis and use it to make and evaluate your decisions.

My soldier friend was feeling pretty guilty when I talked to him. He said, "I should have noticed men were looking down on us from the roof tops before we entered that street. I was on the radio talking to headquarters when I should have been assessing the situation."

Numerous good endeavors have ultimately failed due to the lack of a situational analysis. I challenge you be like "the men of Issachar, who understood the times and knew what Israel should do…" (1 Chronicles 12:32, NIV 1984). You will avoid getting ambushed.

CHAPTER 16
EMINENT OR PREEMINENT

How in the world did I get this old? My life is past its mid-point, maybe even way beyond it. My dad had a heart attack at age 61 while visiting us in Kenya, and he died four years later after acquiring malaria when he and mom returned for a visit. No guarantees of three score and ten or longer.

Birthdays are good in a number of ways. If you stop having them, you are dead. Okay, I'm not dead yet. That's good news! People give you gifts, but those drop off as you get older. Maybe because they often give you things you don't need or want. They somehow realize that, so they stop giving gifts.

Birthdays are a great time for reflection as well. Reflection is something all of us who live such busy lives should do more. I know I get so busy running to do the next thing that I don't spend enough time considering if the next thing is worth doing. Not that I'm doing bad things. Those things, thank God, are almost always easy to discern.

The challenge is in distinguishing the eminent from the preeminent. What falls under the heading of "important" and what should be listed as "most important?" Yeah. That is an important, I mean most important, question!

And it is a question that should be asked periodically of every area of our lives—our work, our family, and our personal spiritual walk with God.

I recently spent an hour writing a long detailed e-mail to a CMDA member who had questions about healthcare reform. It was a very poor investment of my "lifetime." As I thought back, I realized it would have been more important to have spent that time creating a resource that I could give to everyone with questions. Most importantly, I could have invested an hour in having a webinar and invited all CMDA members to log in online to discuss this issue.

I need to weed the hill that goes down to the woods behind my house. During the last few years, I've invested lots of time planting vinca, a ground cover, on a bare hill I can't mow. It was important for erosion, aesthetics, and crowding out weeds.

But my important project hasn't done anything but control erosion. It doesn't look good because of all the weeds that grow among the vinca anyway. Jody and I spend many hours weeding that hill each season. If I had done the most important thing, I would have paid the cost in money and time, put down landscaping fabric, and then planted the vinca. Now I ask myself, "Do I really want to weed this hill the rest of my life?"

That is a mundane example about doing the important, the eminent, instead of the preeminent. If I had done the preeminent with the hill, I would have time tonight to write an article for a magazine that could touch thousands of people. Or I could spend some great time with my family. Or I could go trout fishing. Standing in a river casting a fly is a perfect time for thinking and restoration.

Deciding what is eminent or preeminent is imperative for busy missionaries and their families. There are so many things to do, so many people vying for your time, and so many opportunities.

I have a mental grid that helps me discern (at least some of the time!) what to do. Maybe the questions I ask myself will help you as well.

1. Do I have the skills, abilities, and passion to do this? If not, is it worth the investment of my time to develop it?
2. Is there someone better suited to delegate this to or teach how to do it?
3. Are my motivations biblical? Am I doing this to fulfill biblical mandates of how I should invest my life or am I doing it for fame, power, or fortune?

- God's primary concern is bringing the lost to Christ, discipling them, and turning them into soul winners.
- My primary responsibilities are to God, my family, and then my ministry.
4. How many people will this affect?
    - Am I fishing or teaching people to fish?
    - Will there be a ripple effect?
5. Is there a more efficient way to accomplish this goal that will have a wider impact or a longer effect?
6. Is it worth the "lifetime" I will have to invest to accomplish it?
7. Are there better investments of my time?

Applying these questions can lead to minor and major changes. You may be investing all your time in medicine and not doing ministry. Maybe you are too focused on procedures and not people building. Maybe you need to focus your medical ministry more to help the church bring people to Christ and disciple people.

For Dr. Tom Hale, a missionary surgeon to Nepal, these types of questions moved him from the eminent of providing surgery to the preeminent of writing a commentary on the entire Bible in the local language and writing books to influence people into missions.

For Susan Carter, a young missionary nurse, these questions moved her from hospital nursing and midwifery to starting a community health program that now reaches more than one million people regularly.

For the fifty-six doctors and spouses who went through CMDA's "Completing Your Call" course over a two-year period, it moved everyone back into practice, but doing it in a new and more effective ministry mode.

No matter how old you are, you are getting older. Your "lifetime" is being spent. Are you making preeminent investments?

CHAPTER 17
THE ART OF RUNNING A MEETING

Meetings are a necessary "evil" that must be mastered. They can consume way too much of your team's time and effort. If you have a meeting with eight senior staff for an hour, you have taken away a person's full day of productivity during the time you met. Don't get me wrong, you have to have some meetings. But you should first remember these four principles to keep meetings:

As Rare As Possible
Since meetings consume time, set the goal to have less sit down meetings and ruthlessly pursue replacing them with better alternatives. Look at the meetings you presently schedule. Are they needed? Are they accomplishing what you intend? Which ones can you eliminate and accomplish your goals in other ways?

> *Tip:* I hate when progress is held up waiting for a meeting or a decision to be made, so we do lots of "meetings on the fly." If I have a problem patient, I may do a "sidewalk consultation" or get the key people around the patient's bed to make a decision quickly. So do the same in management. Quickly call the needed people together and decide what needs to be done. This keeps things moving.

Involving As Few People As Possible
Meetings often have people at them who are not really needed. They are there because you don't want them to be left out. That is a big waste of productivity. Figure out some other way to keep them in the loop.

> *Tip:* Do a survey of those in regular meetings and ask questions

like: Do you wish you didn't have to come to this meeting? What are better, more efficient ways to accomplish your job description?

As Brief As Possible
If you are not careful, people arrive late, personal discussions start, and your meeting takes ten to fifteen minutes longer to get underway. Insist everyone arrive five minutes early and start the meeting exactly on time whether everyone is there or not. What is expected is what gets done.

Avoid letting meetings get off track. At a recent board meeting during the Executive Session, someone reverted us back to a topic we discussed earlier during the regular session and we found ourselves talking general board business without the CEO in attendance. This is a big "no-no." I had to interrupt and get us back on track.

Continue to ask, "How can we accomplish our meeting goals in less time?" Set a time limit to each meeting. My rule is no meeting should last more than an hour and many should be scheduled for much less time than that. I was recently at the CMDE conference in Thailand, and noted the teaching sessions were shortened to forty-five minutes. I asked why, and they related studies showing that teachers at hour-long meetings spent fifteen minutes telling jokes and personal anecdotes not substantive to the topic.

> *Tip:* Have stand up meetings where you don't sit down. Studies show they take one-third to one-half the time. Some teams such as those at ward shift changes have stand up "Scrums" each day that only last five to ten minutes to relate problems and status reports from those leaving to those arriving. Stand up gatherings can work well for many types of meetings.

As Focused As Possible
It takes time for people to get on track. The more often you "jump tracks," the more time you spend regaining momentum. Keep the meeting focused on what is important and stick to it. Keep everyone's nose to the grindstone by recapping discussions, asking questions, and letting everyone know you want their input to be concise. You may want to use a white board if you are brainstorming.

> *Tip:* Don't let one person dominate the discussions or go on and on. Solicit opinions from those not contributing. Don't hesitate to creatively interrupt those not getting to their point by saying something like, "How would you summarize what you are saying in one sentence?" If a person is a perennial problem, meet with them between meetings to constructively discuss how they can better contribute.

There is more to the art of running a good meeting than these four principles. You can take some practical steps to make your meetings run smoother. Here is what I recommend:

Prepare For It
Clearly communicate what issues are being covered in the meeting, where it will be held, and how long it is expected to last. Send background materials, handouts, previous minutes, and other materials as far in advance as possible. Include an itemized draft agenda and solicit other items they may want to discuss. Ask each participant to review all the meeting materials before the meeting begins. Also, don't forget to ask for prayer if major changes or new endeavors are being considered.

Preparation may also include pre-meeting discussions with important stakeholders to uncover issues that need to be addressed or to get buy in from an influential attender.

> *Tip:* Don't use valuable meeting time reporting individual attendee's activities. Before our monthly senior staff meeting, each person circulates a status report on their area of responsibilities that answers three simple questions: Your Progress? Your Problems? Your Plans? Each staff member is expected to review those reports before the meeting. That way we can focus our meeting on problem solving, coordination of efforts, and envisioning.

Organize It
Meeting agendas are a crucial road map to success. Start out with prayer, approve the minutes if you have them from the last meeting, and then approve the agenda. Follow this with "Old Business" which are items you have previously dealt with. This may be unfinished business or a report on the results of a decision made. Follow this

with "New Business" which are items being brought up for the first time. Add a section for "Any Other Business" where last minute items can be addressed. These should be rare if you have organized and prepared well.

> *Tip:* In my senior staff meetings, I always add a section to the agenda for "Discussion" and include items that need envisioning, long-range planning, or a broad overview of effectiveness. I don't want us to get so involved in the details during our meetings that we don't take time to look at the big picture. It is dangerous to be so close to the trees that you can't see the forest. Discussion is the time for broad questions like: What is the reputation of our medical ministry? How can we improve staff morale? If we were starting this area of ministry over again, what would we do differently?

Time It
If you are having a longer meeting like a board meeting or have a history of not getting done within the time limits you have announced, time each item on your agenda. This gives you early warning that you are behind and encouragement if you are ahead. It helps keep the leader on track and attenders focused on moving forward.

> *Tip:* If you are having problems projecting accurate times, have the meeting secretary note how much time is being used on each agenda item. Afterwards, sit down and review the timing. If you went over the allotted time, was it because you didn't move things along well or you projected too little time? That will help you do better at the next meeting. If you don't allow adequate time for discussion, your attenders will get frustrated.

> *Tip:* Use committees to save time on large agendas. Put board members on committees where they can use their expertise and meet before the general meeting. For example, you may have a Finance Committee, Governance Committee, and a Strategic Planning Committee. Each committee needs a staff member assigned to assist it. Committees make recommendations to the board and do the board's work. Board committees have no control over staff. You can also assign smaller task forces or ad hoc committees to bring recommendations to a staff group.

Control It
Good meeting leaders encourage the airing of different viewpoints and healthy debate. You want to have your organizational wagon pulled by spirited horses, but you can't let them run out of control. Step in quickly to quell personal attacks, manage negative conflict, identify areas of commonality, and make sure issues are resolved. Make it known to your staff that you welcome freewheeling discussion, but each team member is expected to support the decision once it is made.

It is divisive for board or staff members to leave a meeting and start politicking their own personal positions with others. It is even worse to break confidentiality. If you are discussing confidential matters, let everyone know what they are and that they should not be discussed with others.

> *Tip:* Try to get as much consensus on important decisions as possible, but take formal votes if you are having formal board or similar meetings. If everyone has to agree for a decision to be made, then an individual member can veto any decision. That is not healthy and can incapacitate progress. It is also not healthy to move forward if a board is seriously divided on an important issue. You may need to step in and table the item. Collect more information if needed or ask people to pray about the issue before the next meeting.

Document It
The more complex or long the meeting, the more you need formal minutes. They remind you of the decisions made, serve as an official record, and function as a starting point for the next meeting. They are very useful to give to those who weren't able to attend, but need to know what occurred.

> *Tip:* Review the minutes of the meeting before they are circulated. Your minute taker may have misunderstood something, given something more prominence than it deserved, or explained something poorly. You can correct the minutes before they are circulated. For groups with fiduciary responsibilities like a hospital board, the minutes are legal documents and need to be signed and kept in a secure place.

Tip: For official minutes, I like to use a readily understood numbering system. For example the first minute may be 9/3/12–1 New Hospital Ward. The numbers denote the meeting of the ninth day of March 2012 and this is the first minute of that meeting. When you are doing old business, you can add after the minute title, (Ref: 16/11/10 -5). That means to find the old minute on this topic refer to the fifth minute of meeting from November 16, 2010.

Summarize It

Take a few minutes at the end of the meeting to summarize decisions, assignments that have been given, and items requiring more discussion. This makes sure everyone heard the same thing and you are going to move forward. The most common critique of meetings is that they lasted too long and didn't accomplish anything. Meetings are a waste of time if they don't contribute to progress. Summarizing emphasizes what was accomplished and makes sure momentum is maintained.

Tip: It is a good practice to pull out "Action Items" from the minutes and restate them at the conclusion of the meeting. Make sure these action items note who has the responsibility to take action and when that action must be accomplished.

Okay, meetings aren't "evil" and there is a place for them. They can only be great meetings if you master leading them to produce significant results in a reasonable amount of time. If you apply these principles and practical steps, you can be a "Master of the Art of Leading a Meeting."

PART 5
BUDGETS AND FINANCES

CHAPTER 18
BUDGETING AND THE MISSIONARY DOCTOR

Yes, I'm going to sleep too! No single word makes me more lethargic than the word budgeting. It works better than Ambien! Yet, budgeting is like the correct insulin dosage for a Type 1 diabetic. If you don't figure it out, you are going to have both short- and long-term problems.

If you already have a budgeting process in place, you probably can improve upon it; if not, these suggestions will help you start a process that will serve you well.

Develop Your Budget
The first step is to decide how to develop your budget by setting up income and expense centers. What organizational level will give you enough information to make good decisions without being too burdensome?

One principle I adhere to is to follow the administrative structure down to the level where I want individual staff to be accountable. Usually that is down to the department level. Some departments may only have expenditures and you don't monitor their income since it comes in globally through patient fees. On the other hand, you may want to allocate income to departments so you see which ones are profitable or not.

The other principle is that an area usually needs to be a cost center if its employees have the authority to spend funds. With that authority, they need to know where their limits are and have a way to monitor how they are doing. Name each cost center and enter it onto a spreadsheet.

Review Previous Expenses

Next, you need to attach an income and/or expense projection to each cost center for the first year. To accomplish this, you need to first decide the individual budget lines that each cost center will have—salaries, benefits, supplies, equipment, postage, repairs, etc. You standardize these for your organization so each cost center uses the same naming of budget lines though they may not have amounts to enter into every line. (That way the salary budget from every department can roll up into the global salary cost for the entire organization.) Your projections are based on your experience from the last complete financial year. This is a significant undertaking, but it is easier in subsequent years because you keep financial records in the proper budget format.

Make Your Budget Assumptions

For a new budget, global decisions will affect everyone involved in the budgeting process. Will a cost of living increase in salaries be included in the next budget and what amount will that percentage be? Will there be merit raises in the next year? If so, what range of increases will be allowed and what is the total amount to be allocated for this? What changes will there be in non-salary costs for each employee—health benefits, insurance, government taxes, etc.? How much is income going up because of an increase in fees? What are the projections on outpatient and inpatient admissions? Is the average bill amount going up or down? All such budget items, predetermined by the central administration, must be included when budget worksheets are given to the individuals completing departmental budgets.

Bottoms Up

Get the employees who implement the budget involved in establishing it. In other words, the budget process should start from the ground up, so that the person with the most intimate knowledge of the resources and needs of an income and/or expense area is involved in forming that particular part of the budget proposal.

For example, the information technology center supervisor is going to have the best knowledge of the personnel, supply, equipment, and vendor needs of the department and what each item will cost. For this reason, each cost center's budget items are distributed on a spreadsheet showing the amount spent or received to date in the current financial year as well as a projection of what that amount will be at the end of the financial year. On the same line should be a column showing this year's budget and a column for next year's budget projection.

Budget Line Justifications
It is not enough to pick a number out of thin air that changes the previous year's expense or income budget, either up or down, without justifying it with a short rationale in a note column.

Budget Roll Up
Sections of the budget are rolled up to the senior staff level. All items are reviewed to make sure the budget line projection is reasonable and accomplishes the stated mission, goals, and objectives of your organization.

Budget Balancing
Someone has to do the final roll up review and be the arbitrator. This year at CMDA, we had hundreds of thousands of dollars in projected expenses more than projected income. Some things were obvious to cut. I wasn't getting a CMDA-owned Porsche to drive! (Just kidding!) But the red pencil came out and certain things that were not needed or were over budgeted for were simply adjusted or eliminated. Each department head was brought in to discuss the changes in the budget and to look at other less obvious areas being considered for adjustments. Sometimes the final arbitrator had to make a decision about what was more important than something else that was genuinely needed.

More Than Balancing
It is not enough to balance the budget. An organization needs to budget for a cushion to ensure adequate reserves against a shortfall, and to build up some cash reserves for emergencies or bad years. You may want to pick an amount or a percentage of your overall budget. The smaller that amount, the harder it is to end the year in the black because the "target" is so small.

Budget Approval
The overall budget needs to be reviewed and approved by the board

or other supervisory body that holds fiduciary responsibility for the organization before the new budget year begins.

Budget Line Transfers
No matter how well you budget, you will not project everything correctly. Some things will cost less than projected and other areas will cost more. It is a good policy to allow savings in one place in the budget to cancel out short falls in other areas within limits. For example, Global Health Outreach is a major budget category. We place no limits on how budget income and expense lines can be adjusted as long as the overall department budget meets its bottom line projections. Between major budget centers, the administration is allowed by the board to shift up or down 10 percent as long as the entire budget's bottom line remains constant. If we need to go outside those limits, we need to get board approval.

Monitoring
A well-prepared budget is a tool to guide spending and monitor your financial health. You can have the fanciest blood pressure cuff in the world, but it does no good if you don't use it. A budget is only helpful if there is a monthly trial balance that is reviewed in comparison to the budget. If income is significantly behind budget projections, you may need to focus on increasing income or decreasing expenses. If a cost center is over budget, there is time to address that with the decision maker in that cost center or look for expense savings in other areas to offset it.

Budgeting is a long and laborious process. Without it, you cannot make good organizational decisions, plan for the future, or avoid financial crises. If you are just starting a budgeting process, find an institution like yours with a good budget process in place. Visit them, ask for the electronic file for the budget categories they use, and ask their financial director what they would do with their own process to improve it. Taking time to learn from others will save you lots of time and headaches.

CHAPTER 19
DISSOCIATIVE THINKING

In my carnality, I hate money! Okay, I know that sounds weird so let me break it down. "For the love of money is the root of all kinds of evil" (1 Timothy 6:10, NLT). The Bible clearly teaches this, and I believe it. Christine Stead slyly made that same point when she said, "If all the rich people in the world divided up their money among themselves there wouldn't be enough to go around."

People will pursue wealth and the feeling of power it gives to the detriment of everything with real value.

George Bernard Shaw overstated his point when he quipped, "Lack of money is the root of all evil," but he gets much closer to the reason for my love/hate relationship with "filthy lucre." I hate money because there are so many good things in ministry I cannot do for the lack of it!

I bet you battle the same feelings. Your life is full of, "If we just had the money, we could...." I bet lots of words would fit into that blank space—build a nursing school, start a residency program, improve immunization coverage, hire more nurses or a national doctor, and many more.

The lists I would write to fill that vacant space would be different, but just as long as yours. That's why I have been mulling over money lately. I think I made some progress on this issue that you might find helpful.

I serve as the vice chair of the board of Asbury University, my alma mater that was called Asbury College until recently. Former National

Commander of the Salvation Army Israel Gaither gave a rousing challenge at chapel inaugurating the name change, noting that the name change was not a celebration of past accomplishments but a new start—an opportunity for greater ministry and influence than ever before. Everyone, including me, jumped to our feet in a standing ovation as he concluded.

Afterwards, I went to a meeting of the board development committee that I serve on. This committee is supposed to help the administration find the funding needed to start new construction on buildings and develop new programs. After we heard reports, we moved into a brainstorming session. The bottom line was similar to the bottom line of your ministry: the university did not have a constituency with enough wealth to accomplish all it needed to do.

As someone said, the definition of lunacy is doing the same thing over and over again, thinking you will get a different result. What we usually do is spend our brainstorming time tweaking what we did in the past which only marginally increases our financial support.

And then a board member, a retired businessman from a large corporation, related doing the same thing at his company until a new leader decided they needed to change their whole pattern of thinking. They should not spend all their efforts figuring out how to increase sales 5 to 10 percent in the next year. Instead, they needed to disassociate from the progress curve they were on with all its focus on incremental improvement.

They needed to step outside that "boxed-in" approach and instead ask, "What could we do to take us to a whole new level of success?" What could dramatically change the company's future and move its growth curve to a much steeper slope?

It's the kind of dissociative thinking Thomas Edison did. He didn't spend all of his time trying to figure out how to make gas lights work more efficiently or burn brighter. He stepped away from the concept of improvement and created the light bulb, the first phonograph, and the first movie projector.

Get the picture? (Pun intended) So let's return to money issues to do a little dissociative thinking and consider some examples. I suspect you have major projects that need to be done and a list of donors who don't have the resources to accomplish many of them. How can you find a better source of income?

Indiana Wesleyan University used to be the small, unknown Marion Bible College with great financial needs. Dissociative thinking led them outside the box to begin providing distance learning via the internet and satellite campuses. Someone smartly noted that the profit margins were much higher when you didn't have to build dormitories and cafeterias while running sports programs for students. They now have 12,000 day students all across the Midwest and have grown their residential student body to 4,000 with the proceeds resulting in a state of the art campus. Now the university has much more impact.

Perhaps your ministry could reorganize to do the same thing, not stopping what you are currently doing, but expanding it based on a total new income generating outreach.

In our development meeting at Asbury, we realized we weren't going to develop dramatically different fundraising results by approaching the same supporters of the college. In large part, they were supporting the school to the best of their ability. Dissociative thinking led us to the conclusion that we would reach a "hinge point," if we could find one or two very wealthy donors who would not just support a particular project but become champions for the entire university. Wealthy people have wealthy friends they can recruit to help. Another small college recruited a very wealthy board member who then recruited two or three more. With only 600 students, that school successfully completed a $50 million dollar capital campaign, more than ever dreamed possible just a few years before. The vast majority of the money came from those wealthy board members and their friends.

So here is my challenge to you. I want you to become a dissociative thinker! No, I'm not talking about the medical disorder of depersonalization. I want you to get together with some of your most creative thinkers and ask yourself, "What could we do that would take us to a whole new level of financial support or ministry effectiveness?" While you are brainstorming, forget those things that are behind and press forward to what God has in store.

Get outside the limits of what your mind says is possible, seek God's wisdom, and pray. Do some "dissociative thinking." Who knows what may happen?

PART 6
PERSONNEL MATTERS

CHAPTER 20
YOUR MOST NEEDED RESOURCE

The greatest need in medical missions today is long-term personnel. Without competent, compassionate doctors, nurses, and other personnel who know the language, culture, and needs of the local people, mission/church health programs will not last long. Career missionaries are the fulcrum upon which short-term personnel leverage their efforts. They design the programs, construct the buildings, work with the national church, maintain government relationships, and earn the trust of the local people. They are experts in contextualizing the gospel and presenting it to the local people.

That is why CMDA set a goal to increase the number of career medical missionaries by 25 percent over the next five years with a multifaceted initiative. We are enhancing our efforts to get medical students and residents on rotations overseas. Last year, more than sixty students and thirty residents received financial assistance to be involved in these overseas rotations, and we motivated hundreds more. We set a goal of doubling the number of missionaries we financially assist in the years ahead. Scholarships average $500 for students and $1,000 for residents.

It is unlikely a young person would become a mechanic if they had never looked under a vehicle's hood. It is also unlikely that they will go into missions unless they have seen what it is like firsthand. God uses such experiences to call individuals into career service as He takes them out of their comfort zones and gets their attention.

Many first and second year medical and dental students, as well as premed college and nursing students, long to shadow missionary doctors and nurses. During a presentation, I had to tell 200 such students at Indiana Wesleyan University that I didn't know of a mission health facility that would take them. I know what you are thinking. The housing, feeding, and time required to deal with these students is time consuming and they can't be of much help since they lack clinical skills. But the more basic issue is that the earlier you get young people committed to medical missions, the more likely they are to end up overseas.

I still remember shadowing Dr. Steury after my junior year in college. Ernie and Sue had to put a couple of their kids on the couch so I would have a bedroom, plus I was an extra place setting at every meal. But as I watched this humble, competent doctor share devotions at the table, perform a complicated surgery, fix a badly broken hospital generator, get up at night to take care of patients, and win people to Christ, I was dramatically impacted. A nurse taught me to pass instruments in surgery and I even got to deliver my first baby. I was hooked. Not only did God call me back to Tenwek, but I found inspiration for the long road ahead.

We should get future missionary colleagues overseas during college and also continue to get them back at every stage of their training. For physicians, that means during medical school and residency. You have to continue to stoke the fire to ward off the chilling effects of "professionalization."

CMDA is also focusing more efforts on informing practicing doctors about second-career opportunities through our publications, websites, and placement services. I encourage you to let us know your personnel needs in the short- or long-term. It is helpful to have a central location where people can learn about your needs.

We are working hard to get graduate doctors and their families overseas through Global Health Outreach on one of our short-term trips each year or through World Medical Mission to serve for longer periods. The Global Missions Health Conference in Louisville, Kentucky, is growing by leaps and bounds. On average, more than 2,400 attend, including 600 students, who visit 120 exhibits, attend some of the 80 workshops, network, and attend inspiring plenaries. You need to plan to attend this conference during the second week of November when you are on home assignment.

What can you do to increase the number of career medical missionaries joining you in service? First of all, pray to the Lord of the harvest that He will send more laborers into the field. It is the most essential thing. Secondly, get intentional about recruiting co-laborers. Let me break it down into some practical steps.

Build a Database of Prospects

Create a subset of your database with fields noting those in practice or training. Note their field of training, how far along they are, and any personal information about them. Create a short communication piece—besides your regular prayer letter—to send to this group, sharing interesting medical stories, insights into the challenges you face, information about your institution, and opportunities to visit during training.

Recruit During Your Home Assignment Time

Often on furlough, you are going from church to church to raise funds. Set aside time in your schedule to spend time and effort where you can raise co-workers. Speak at Christian colleges, professional schools, residencies, and graduate doctor groups. Focus your message on the spiritual characteristics that God wants to nurture in individuals' lives so they will be missionaries wherever they serve. Illustrate principles like self-denial, obedience, sacrifice, boldness, compassion, caring for the poor, and evangelism with gripping personal stories from your work, personal experiences, and family life. Challenge those in training to visit and spend time with you.

Let the Center for Medical Missions know of your schedule, and they will get the word out to our regional and area directors so you can have a chance to speak at some student or graduate chapters.

Improve Your Short-Termer's Experience

I've seen short-term staff poorly supported, isolated, and even abused. Poor orientation, lack of on-the-job training, little exposure to the community, poor communication, no spiritual ministry opportunities, and too much night call are just a short list of some of the problems I've seen. It amazed me when I headed World Medical Mission that some doctors were never even invited into a missionary's home, though they had paid their way, reduced their practice income, and given generously of their talents at a hospital for a month.

Here is my ten-point checklist for ensuring a great short-term experience for students and doctors:

1. Prepare the Way - There is a great deal of anxiety for individuals and families going overseas. Take time to communicate with your visitors before they arrive. Create pre-trip information materials and suggest resources to read. Use a group like World Medical Mission for graduates to help you handle all the details. Appoint a contact person from your mission team, but make sure one person with the same type of training contacts those coming by e-mail beforehand. Creating a website for your ministry with lots of pictures and information can be very helpful.

2. Optimize Orientation - Make newcomers feel welcome. Facilitate introductions. Take them on a tour of your facilities. Create an orientation booklet with medicine lists, normal therapies for common diseases, key policies, information on dealing with national staff, culture tips, maps, communication information, and much more. It takes time, but it will save you more time in the long run. Update this orientation booklet regularly.

3. Appoint a Mentor - Ask one of your missionaries to take each short-term volunteer or family under their wing. That should include professional and personal time together. The goal is to give a picture of what it is like to be a missionary. The key is to let the individual or family spend time with missionaries as they live their daily lives. Take the volunteers to church, invite them over for a meal, take them to visit national friends in the community, check with them at the end of the day to see how they are doing, and answer their many questions.

4. Be Wise in Work Assignments - Use but don't abuse your volunteers. Don't give them more night call than is normal. Don't give them more responsibility than they can reasonably handle for their level of training. Increase or lessen responsibility based on how they are doing. Give them time off like career staff. You may not be able to put a student or resident exclusively in their area of interest, but make sure they get some exposure to areas of interest. Make sure volunteers have proper backup to ensure quality patient care. Let them spend as much time as possible with

career healthcare personnel as they diagnose, teach, and treat. Much of the art of what you do is better caught than taught.

5. Don't Let Your Volunteers Get Isolated - Guesthouses and apartments are nice but they also can easily lead to isolation. Without career staff readily available to answer questions and explain policies, a clique of volunteers can develop. One bad apple can affect the whole barrel and before you know it, you can have a "them versus us" mentality and unhappy volunteers.

6. Have Some Fun - All work and no play leads to burnout and dissatisfaction. Invite volunteers over for a video or game night. Take them on a trip. Visit a historical site. Celebrate a holiday. Involve them in one of your hobbies. Exercise or play a sport together.

7. Make Sure They Get to Know the Local People - Ask national staff members to invite them into their homes. Let them go to outlying clinics. Set up visits to local churches. Help them learn the local language and culture by loaning out resources.

8. Give Opportunities to Do Ministry - Let them speak in chapel if you are in a hospital or share in a local church. If you have chaplains, let them spend some time ministering to patients or going on home follow-up visits. We used to have visitors speak in chapel with our head chaplain translating. He filled in the voids in the visitor's message so well that patients often came to Christ. Those experiences were the highlights visitors talked about for weeks.

9. Formally Debrief - Take time to have those who worked closely with the volunteers debrief them. What went well? What could have been done better? How did God work in their life during their time there? What are their thoughts about long-term missionary service? If appropriate, tell them that you would love to have them come back long-term or sometime later during their training. Express your appreciation for what they did. Pray with them and make sure you have current contact information for follow-up. Jot down the essence of the conversation in a short report to file and share with your leadership. You may want to assign an overall rating to each person to prioritize your follow-up.

10. Follow-up, Follow-up, and Follow-up - Most missionaries are busy and don't follow-up with volunteers after they return home. That's a big mistake. Personalize communication to your top prospects. Assign the person who developed the closest relationship with the volunteer to nurture it. Keep them updated on your work, ask for advice, send them follow-up information on patients they took care of, and request their help in finding supplies, equipment, and medicine. Your goal is to keep them involved in your ministry and get them back to work with you again short- or long-term. Visit them during your home assignment and continue to let them know you would love to have them back. Get them to your mission's national meeting.

Recruiting career missionaries is a long process, but it is worth the investment of time and energy. You can do it better than your headquarters' staff. With prayer, good planning, and attention to the details, God will supply the colleagues you need.

CHAPTER 21
CONFLICT RESOLUTION

My sister and brother-in-law arrived on the mission field in South America while I was still in medical school. By the time Jody and I were ready for service, they had finished their first term and were "experienced" missionaries. I can only remember one piece of advice he gave as we prepared to head overseas, but it was a jewel. He said, "Dave, your greatest blessings will come from your relationships with other missionaries. They will also be your greatest source of conflict and tension." At that time, I thought all missionaries were super Christians who had received their heavenly haloes early!

After arriving on the field, it didn't take me long to learn the truth of my brother-in-law's prophecy. In fact, the possibility of missionary conflict is amplified because you don't get to choose your colleagues and are forced to work, worship, play, and live in close proximity. The potential for problems compounds because you live in a high pressure environment where night call, patient loads, and administrative duties make you even more interdependent. For example, if someone goes on vacation or is not carrying the load, you are obligated to pick up extra duties.

Problems are further aggravated by the usual overdose of work, limited staff (if someone gets mad and leaves, you get to do that job until the mission finds a replacement), and often a lack of pastoral care. It is a guaranteed recipe for resentment, anger, bitterness, and even the occasional knockdown, drag out fight. (I could share illustrative stories, but I won't in order to protect the guilty!)

I want to share some advice on conflict resolution drawn in part from one of CMDA's grandchildren. We helped birth the Christian Legal Society many years ago, which later created and spun off Peacemaker Ministries. This ministry produced an incredible number of great resources on this topic that you can check out at *www.peacemaker.net*. I used their Christian mediation and arbitration services soon after taking the helm at CMDA in a difficult situation we had with another Christian organization. They did such a great job that we routinely use the group for mediation and arbitration in all of our contracts.

Let's start by learning how to deal with conflicts with others, move to helping others resolve conflict, and then talk about prophylaxis to reduce the incidence of future conflict. These principles are well worth the time to learn and practice as they can be applied to work, marriage, family, church, and friendship situations.

Here is the situation. You have a colleague who is outgoing, personable, and loves people. He loves traveling, meeting new people, and interacting with nationals. The problem is that he has trouble sticking with the grind of the heavy workload at your hospital. He is eager and ready to make clinic visits, take visiting staff out to the community, go on a business trip, get involved on a variety of mission committees that require extensive time away, and accept enumerable preaching opportunities. When he is gone, he always seems to find a reason to extend the length of his time away.

At first you just picked up the extra load, but then it became a source of irritation. You complained to your spouse about it. She threw some fuel on the fire by telling you that you were justified in being upset and she was tired of you having to do more than your share of the work. It was time away from her and the children.

After that your irritation embers burst into anger flames. A few sparks flew as you share your "concern" via some sarcastic comments to others on the subject of his "lack of a good work ethic." Unbeknownst to you, some of those words travel back to him, lighting his fire. He retaliates by telling visiting staff about your workaholic personality that "doesn't really care about people like he does."

You learn about some of his comments and that throws even more gasoline to your fire. Your anger bursts into bitterness. Your communication becomes even shorter and more stilted when you talk to him. Your wives avoid each other. The other missionaries start picking sides. You begin to think the best thing might be to get out of this mess and return to the U.S.

If this isn't your scenario, you probably experienced something similar to it on this or another issue. You traveled down the road from irritation, to anger, to bitterness, to broken relationships, and even to a desire to punish someone.

Where do you begin to get out of such a mess? First start with your own heart's desires. James 4:1-3 says,

> "What causes fights and quarrels among you? Don't they come from your desires that battle within you? You want something but don't get it. You kill and covet, but you cannot have what you want. You quarrel and fight. You do not have, because you do not ask God. When you ask, you do not receive, because you ask with wrong motives, that you may spend what you get on your pleasures" (NIV 1984).

The desires of our hearts are the wellspring of our conflicts. It usually bubbles up from a belief that our "rights" of justice and autonomy are not being recognized and respected. Sometimes that is the case, but either way the first step is to put your desires on the altar before trying to work through the conflict.

You need to conclude that your happiness and fulfillment are not held in someone else's hand, but are found in God alone (Psalm 73:25). For Christians, the statement, "I could be happy if…" should not be in our vocabulary. Our fulfillment is found in Christ alone and He uses conflict to teach and mature us as He says in James 1:2-4:

> "Consider it a sheer gift, friends, when tests and challenges come at you from all sides. You know that under pressure, your faith-life is forced into the open and shows its true colors. So don't try to get out of anything prematurely. Let it do its work so you become mature and well-developed, not deficient in any way" (MSG).

Understanding the wellspring of your anger is the first step to reconciliation as you ask God to deal with you before you deal with others.

The second stem is to ask God to cleanse your heart of bitterness and give you a genuine love for the person you have conflict with. I remember when Dr. Steury and I dealt with a difficult situation where someone treated him very badly. He had every reason to be angry and upset, but he wasn't. He told me why. He said, "Dave, I've learned if I genuinely pray for God's best for the person I'm having a problem with, it changes my attitude towards them. I don't ask for God to change them. I ask God to overflow my heart with love for them."

Paul learned this lesson and personally applied it. He said in 1 Corinthians 4:12, "When they call us names, we say, 'God bless you'" (MSG). Christ summed up what we should do when we have conflict with someone in Luke 6:27-28:

> "To you who are ready for the truth, I say this: Love your enemies. Let them bring out the best in you, not the worst. When someone gives you a hard time, respond with the energies of prayer for that person" (MSG).

In 1 John 4:19-21, John reiterates and tells us that loving those who treat us badly is not an option to consider but a command to follow:

> "…First we were loved, now we love. He loved us first. If anyone boasts, 'I love God,' and goes right on hating his brother or sister, thinking nothing of it, he is a liar. If he won't love the person he can see, how can he love the God he can't see? The command we have from Christ is blunt: Loving God includes loving people. You've got to love both" (MSG).

Wow! You just thought you were doing well if you could tolerate that person, but God set the standard. He loved us when we were unlovable. Because He loved us, we are commanded and also enabled to love the one who harmed us.

The other thing we tend to do when we have a conflict is judge the other person in thought, word, or deed. We criticize, talk behind their back, nitpick, gossip, and coerce them if we have the power to do so. Christ cautions us about this in Luke 6:37, "Don't pick on people, jump on their failures, criticize their faults—unless, of course, you want the same treatment" (MSG).

Note that this verse admits the person in question has failed and is at fault, but this admission doesn't give us the right to step into God's role as judge and jury to condemn them. Does that mean we should just ignore their actions?

The Bible teaches that there is a right and a wrong way to judge. We are commanded not to do it out of contempt, a sense of moral superiority, or bitterness. We may need to confront a situation but we must do so out of a pure motive of seeking that person's good. One type of judging mentally condemns the person to punishment. The other type of judgment realistically sees the situation and tries to restore the relationship. Check out this verse in Matthew 7:4-5:

> "Do you have the nerve to say, 'Let me wash your face for you,' when your own face is distorted by contempt? It's this whole traveling road-show mentality all over again, playing a holier-than-thou part instead of just living your part. Wipe that ugly sneer off your own face, and you might be fit to offer a washcloth to your neighbor" (MSG).

And then in Galatians 6:1, it says, "…If someone falls into sin, forgivingly restore him, saving your critical comments for yourself. You might be needing forgiveness before the day's out" (MSG).

Which brings us to the last bit of soul surgery we need to submit to by our heavenly surgeon. We must unconditionally forgive the person who wronged us, even before they ask for forgiveness. Paul says it more explicitly in Colossians 3:13, "Be even-tempered, content with second place, quick to forgive an offense. Forgive as quickly and completely as the Master forgave you" (MSG).

The standard God set is complete and immediate forgiveness for the hurt someone heaped on us whether they "deserve" it or not. We didn't deserve God's forgiveness but He freely forgave our sins.

Let me give you a practical word of advice at this point. You may need to have personal help in dealing with your anger, bitterness, or even rage. Find a friend you can be completely honest with. Tell that friend how you think and feel about the situation, not in a way to put the focus on the other person but in a way to empty your own heart. Ask them to pray for you that God will give you a generous, overflowing love for the person who offended you and flood your heart with forgiveness. Often just saying how you feel out loud has a wonderful therapeutic effect that can effectively turn the tide as you pray with your friend.

When your attitudes and actions have a godly adjustment, thank Him and rejoice! This is the most important and the hardest thing you need to do in dealing with conflict. You can't control the other person so the only results you are responsible for in resolving the conflict is to get your heart healed and your mind mended to God's way of thinking.

Now, for the next step—dealing with the person you are in conflict with. After you have determined to trust, obey, and imitate Christ in a conflict, how do you move forward in dealing with the person you had a conflict with in a way that will glorify God?

First, you need to "duck" some offenses, and I mean that in both senses of the word! There are some issues that you should avoid dealing with because they don't rise to a level of importance that merits addressing. Ken Sande, the President of Peacemakers, recommends that offenses be overlooked if you can answer "no" to the following questions:

- Is the offense seriously dishonoring God?
- Has it permanently damaged a relationship?
- Is it seriously hurting other people?
- Is it seriously hurting the offender himself?

If it is not a serious offense, imitate a duck and let it roll off your back like drops of water. This may mean ignoring a real offense—someone does not give you credit for the work you are doing, imposed more than your share of the work on you, said something unkind about you to others, and the list goes on. It may or may not be a habitual pattern. Either way you have to decide whether you are going to get upset, take offense, and make an issue out of it.

After years of being in leadership over a wide variety of people, I've learned it is critical to know when and when not to duck. If the situation is affecting the ministry, damaging relationships, causing a poor testimony, or seriously damaging the perpetrator, it must be dealt with. If it is just irritating me, I need to do my duck imitation and forget it. "Smart people know how to hold their tongue; their grandeur is to forgive and forget" (Proverbs 19:11, MSG).

In this same vein, you need to interpret other people's actions in the best light. If you are already upset, it is easy to "interpret" every word or deed in the worst way. When this happens, you filter each thing said or done for hidden motives and meanings. You become anaphylactic in the sense that the smallest imagined offense can set off a huge reaction. You are actively looking for evidence to support your forgone conclusion that this person is in error. Many conflicts would disappear if the person offended would just remove the chip from their shoulder and give the other person the benefit of the doubt.

If there is a serious offense, make sure you are pursuing the right goal, the goal of restoration. It is easy to take Matthew 18:15 out of context when it states, "If your brother sins against you, go and show him his fault, just between the two of you…" (NIV 1984).

I've seen people use this direction to "show him his fault" or justify "getting into someone's face" and telling them exactly what their problem is. That rarely, if ever, works.

Just before this verse is the wonderful story of the shepherd and the lost sheep, a metaphor of how God lovingly seeks to restore us to our relationship with Him. Remember that verse 15 concludes by saying, "If he listens to you, you have won your brother over" (NIV 1984).

Winning your brother over does not mean hitting him over the head with a verbal 2x4! It means acting with gentleness, mercy, and good intent. You want to be winsome! The goal is to not only to renew your relationship but to make it better. If you go to a person to prove them wrong, there is little chance that restoration will take place.

Preparation is essential in making peace. First of all pray for wisdom, humility, and a spirit of grace. It is difficult to know exactly what to say and how to communicate it with love. James 1:5 says, "If you don't know what you're doing, pray to the Father. He loves to help" (MSG).

Like you, I've been in conflicts that make it seem difficult, if not impossible, to pray or know what to say to God. The stress and emotions run high. Pray as it commands in Romans 8:26, "If we don't know how or what to pray, it doesn't matter. He does our praying in and for us, making prayer out of our wordless sighs, our aching groans" (MSG).

You may need to find a friend or two who will pray for you. You don't need to take out all the dirty laundry or even tell them whom you are going to talk to. Just let them know you are dealing with an interpersonal conflict. Like Paul in Ephesians 6:19, you can ask, "Don't forget to pray for me. Pray that I'll know what to say and have the courage to say it at the right time" (MSG).

It is also helpful to plan what you are going to say to the person and even rehearse it in especially difficult situations. It is helpful to tell the person how their actions or words made you feel. They can argue about the facts or try to explain their motives, but they can't challenge the emotions you feel. Think about the person's likely responses and think about how you will respond. Practice will help you learn how to better deal with the situation.

A good filter to put your rehearsal through is to ask yourself, "If this was turned around and this person was coming to me, how would I like to be spoken to? What would I want said?" Don't forget to practice using the right tone. Just think of all the ways you can say, "I love you." It can sound sincere, loving, sarcastic, frivolous, questioning, and even mean depending on the tone and inflection you use. Body language also conveys as much or more than the words you say. Pay attention and rehearse all forms of communication to make sure you are sending the right message.

What about a written communication? It usually doesn't work. It does not have tone, inflection, or body language so it can easily be misinterpreted. It also can easily be passed on to others or excerpted out of context. You can't tailor it to how your words are being received as you can in a live conversation. A good principle to adhere to is to never use a letter or an e-mail to deal with conflict. This type of conflicts requires a personal meeting or at least a phone call.

It is critical to pick the right time and place to talk about the issue. Almost always, talking in private without distractions or interruptions is best. You can pick their ground, neutral ground or your ground. There are good reasons for each depending on the situation. Meeting on their ground puts the person more at ease and you control how long the discussion lasts before you decide to leave, but you can't prevent interruptions or distractions. Your ground may be more threatening to the person you are dealing with, but you can control the environment better. Often neutral ground works the best because neither party is boxed in. You could say something like, "Can you come by for a cup of coffee? There is something I would like to talk to you about."

Okay, you have dealt with your personal feelings before God, are prayed up, have practiced, and found the right place. You've approached this biblically, but it is still easy to worry and fret about what could happen, to be nervous, or even scared.

Rest.

- Rest in the knowledge that you are doing what God told you to do and are striving to please Him. God expects faithful obedience and rewards it, not our success.
- Rest in the fact that the outcome is in His hands and you can't control the other person's reactions. Only God can change people.
- Rest in the assurance that you aren't dealing with this alone because God is with you.

Now carry out your plan. During the conversation remember to:

- Listen.
  - "Answering before listening is both stupid and rude" (Proverbs 18:13, MSG).
- Speak wisely.
  - "Watch the way you talk…Say only what helps, each word a gift" (Ephesians 4:29, MSG).
- Get feedback on the other person's feelings and diffuse any anger with a gentle response.
  - "A gentle response defuses anger, but a sharp tongue kindles a temper-fire" (Proverbs 15:1, MSG).
- Remember it may not all be solved in one conversation.

- "God's servant must not be argumentative, but a gentle listener and a teacher who keeps cool, working firmly but patiently with those who refuse to obey. You never know how or when God might sober them up with a change of heart and a turning to the truth" (2 Timothy 2:24-25, MSG).

If the matter is serious and you are unable to get it resolved, you may need to seek a person or two to mediate between the two of you. Ideally, this should be someone both people respect and who has experience in resolving conflicts. "If he won't listen, take one or two others along so that the presence of witnesses will keep things honest, and try again" (Matthew 18:16, MSG). These witnesses can help hold you both accountable, see beyond the rhetoric to the facts, and pray with you both.

Reconciliation requires forgiveness. You need to forgive the person for what they have done to you.

- "Be alert. If you see your friend going wrong, correct him. If he responds, forgive him" (Luke 17:3, MSG).
- "Be gentle with one another, sensitive. Forgive one another as quickly and thoroughly as God in Christ forgave you" (Ephesians 4:32, MSG).
- "Now is the time to forgive this man and help him back on his feet. If all you do is pour on the guilt, you could very well drown him in it" (2 Corinthians 2:7, MSG).

If necessary, you too need to ask for forgiveness for your wrong words, attitudes, thoughts, and actions. Make a conscious decision to be different in the future. Job gives us a great example of this when he said, "I admit I once lived by rumors of you; now I have it all firsthand—from my own eyes and ears! I'm sorry—forgive me. I'll never do that again, I promise! I'll never again live on crusts of hearsay, crumbs of rumor" (Job 42:5-6, MSG). Resolving conflict is hard work and sometimes it does not work despite the fact that you went about it in a biblical manner. What then?

Seek good advice from wise people regarding other approaches to try. If the person won't approach the conflict from a biblical perspective, don't step down to that level. Continue thinking and doing as God mandates. Their intransigence does not give you the right to act unrighteous. Continue to pray for them and God's blessings on their life. Treat them with the most powerful weapon of all, unconditional love.

How do you prevent conflicts or remedy them quickly? Teaching everyone how to recognize and react to conflicts is essential. You may want to take these principles and share them with others or provide them with great resources for individual or group study. Ken Sande's book *The Peacemaker* is available at *www.peacemaker.org*. It is also available as an audio book and workbooks are available for small group studies. There are also resources for families and youth to help others resolve their conflicts.

I want to be a peacemaker. It is one of the key characteristics of good Christian leadership. I hope you too will pursue peace.

CHAPTER 22
ORIENTING SHORT-TERM MEDICAL MISSIONARIES

Short-term missionaries. You can't live without them and sometimes it can be difficult to live with them! Just about the time they become really effective, they head home, leaving you to start another cycle of orientation and training to get the new missionary short-termers up to speed.

At Tenwek, we had more than 50 short-term volunteers each year and they certainly were a godsend. They helped us provide better medical coverage, as well as diagnostic and treatment expertise for conditions that we had difficulty addressing. The best volunteers taught us new things to help us do our jobs better.

In retrospect, I see their greatest contributions more clearly. They freed us up to deal with strategically important issues instead of just the urgent. They gave us the time to plan, build, train, fundraise, and have a greater spiritual ministry. We would never have made the progress we did without their help. We couldn't have progressed far without them. So we housed them. Before we had a guesthouse, Jody and I had visitors in our small home with three kids for nine months out of the year. So we fed them, fed them, and fed them—breakfast, lunch, and supper with no fast food chain restaurants or grocery stores within fifty miles.

Don't get me wrong. I cherish the friendships we developed and our opportunity to model sacrificial living. As my dad once told me, "Dave, you will have as much impact in the states as you will have on the mission field through your lives and testimony." We certainly did, but we didn't realize that some years it would seem like half of America came to visit!

We worked hard to maximize our short-termers' experiences. We wanted it to be a life transforming time that would affect their lives forever, wherever God placed them to serve. It soon became obvious that comprehensive cultural and medical orientation was a recurring and essential component to meeting that goal. After I got some experience under my belt, I sat down and put together some orientation manuals.

One manual focused on orienting to missionary life at our place of service. When was the grocery trip to town? When did the mail go out? What about security issues? When did the electricity go off? Which career missionaries dealt with which issues? When and where were church services? What dress was appropriate? What cultural "dos" and "don'ts" did they need to know?

It took a significant investment of time to put that manual together and continue to update it as we remembered items we forgot to include, but it was well worth the effort. It saved us lots of time and reinforced what we shared verbally. We also appointed each visitor a missionary mentor to encourage them and answer their questions. That became more important as we grew bigger. With so many missionary options, we could select the best mentors for our visitors. You don't want tired and discouraged colleagues dumping their frustrations on short-term volunteers.

The next step was an orientation manual for our healthcare outreach. We actually had two of these manuals. The first manual explained the mechanics of how everything functioned and covered topics like night call, lab ordering, X-ray availability, charting, student and resident roles, ministry opportunities, morning rounds, and dozens of other miscellaneous issues.

The next manual spent time focusing on diagnosis and treatment. What were the appropriate tests to order and what did they cost? What medicines did we have and what diseases were they used for? What were the standard treatment protocols? What were the common diseases we saw and how could they recognize them?

One thing included in these manuals is something you might want to use. It is what I now call:

The Ten Commitments for Short-Term Medical Missionaries
1. I am here to serve, not be served.
2. I know the American philosophy of medicine doesn't apply here.
3. I need to do the best I can for the most people.
4. I accept that I won't have the medicines and equipment I desire and need.
5. I don't know much, so I'm here to learn.
6. I'm not here to change things, so I won't criticize. I recognize that short-term participants don't know the culture, costs, government regulations, and other constraints with which this ministry operates.
7. I'm here to work hard and do more than my share.
8. I will encourage the national and missionary staff.
9. I will happily conform to standards of conduct to protect the testimony of this ministry.
10. I will love and respect the patients I treat.

Perhaps you already have good orientation materials. They are worth their weight in gold. As we continued to adapt our manuals, I would try to get orientation materials from other medical ministries I visited so we could further enhance ours.

The best solution for problems with short-term staff is to prevent problems from ever happening. The best way to send an animated advertisement for your ministry outreach is to send each short-term volunteer home bubbling over with the wonder of their experiences! Who knows, one day they may return as your colleague!

CHAPTER 23
BASIC TRAINING

What would you think of a surgeon who failed to scrub up properly? Oh, he could give you all sorts of reasons—he had too many surgeries, it was an urgent case, or "things aren't that clean here anyway." As a healthcare professional, you could easily predict what would happen. Infectious complications would increase. If you ignore the basics of successful surgery, patients pay the price.

As a doctor, you are extremely busy. Besides providing medical care, you are often called upon to manage the hospital, dispensaries, community health programs, and much more. If you want to be a good manager, you need to pay attention to management basics. If not, sooner or later you are going to pay the price in staff discontent and poor work habits.

Your job as a manager is first to help your staff members understand how important their jobs are. Schedule a time with your hospital's department heads and lead them in a focused discussion on why their jobs are important. Throughout this discussion, use the following questions:

1. In what ways is this facility meeting real needs and doing worthwhile things?
2. What part of your own job contributes to meeting these needs?
3. What part of your job makes special use of your skills, talents, and gifts?
4. What unpleasant but necessary parts of your job are best done by you?

It is best to give the questions out on paper, let each individual personally answer them, and then lead an open discussion where insights are shared. Write their answers on a blackboard or plastic sheet. This lets your staff know that what they shared was important. At the end of the discussion, affirm that:

1. Their jobs are very important.
2. They were created for a purpose.
3. They are not working at the hospital by chance.

Have your supervisors do the same exercise with their employees. This helps every level of the staff understand how their jobs meet the overarching goals of the organization and that they are building God's kingdom. If a job is important, it is worth doing and putting effort into. If your staff members realize that their work is important—whether it is managing the nursing staff, sterilizing instruments, or cleaning the floors—they will be more eager to do it well. They must understand also that you as their leader and the community at large think their work is valuable and needed.

CHAPTER 24
OILING THE GEARS

The devil is not in the details. He is in the midst of a group trying to cause disunity, knowing that when individuals come together so much more can be accomplished for the kingdom. He hates concord, coherence, and congruence or, to put it simply, harmony. Instead he wants to sow discord, dissent, disputes, and divisions to make you and everyone else miserable.

The reason people hate their jobs is either they don't think they are doing something significant or they don't get along with the people they work with. The ongoing friction of being rubbed the wrong way day after day leads to open conflagration or an announcement that someone resigned and took a new job. The more staff turnover you have, the less gets accomplished.

This problem of disunity is more likely to occur in intense work environments, such as healthcare, where good teamwork is crucial to saving the lives of your patients. In that case, it is more than just your staff who suffer. Lack of collaboration and cooperation causes patients to suffer more and even die.

Yet, we are often too busy with our medical or dental duties to pay attention, much less foster solidarity among those we work with and supervise. That is a dangerous and destructive mistake. In the long run, our time and attention will be consumed with trying to put out a forest fire that we could have handled easily with a cup of water when the flame was small.

The key is for your group to work in one accord. What can you do to make this happen?

Put fresh oil in the gears regularly.
I went to a Christian boarding school for high school and didn't own a car until after I graduated from college. Dad let me borrow one of his cars my first summer in college when I sold books door-to-door in Illinois. When I came back in late summer to start another academic year, Dad casually asked, "When did you last change the oil on the car?" I had never maintained a car so my response was a question with a tone of chagrin, "You are supposed to change the oil?"

As a leader, your job is to decrease friction in the motor of your ministry by pouring oil in the gears regularly. Your attitude and interest in your individual staff serves as a great lubricant. Get to know people as personally and intimately as you can. Ask about their families, hobbies, and life outside of the workplace. You want to build a bond between yourself and those you work with. If you have a large staff, you may even need to write down details to keep them all straight. Try to do this with all of your staff members, but especially with your leadership team. Pray for their needs. Send brief notes of encouragement. Think of creative ways to say thank you for their labors and to help them accomplish their work.

Let everyone know the rules of the game.
In the early 1990s, I was invited by the director of Samaritan's Purse-Canada to go to a hockey game while I was in Calgary. I had no idea what "off-sides" or "icing" were, nor did I know the difference between "checking" and "charging." I didn't begin to enjoy the game until he explained what was going on so I understood the rules.

It is the same in the workplace. Each member of your staff needs to know the rules, so you need to outline those rules in a staff policy manual. All employees need to know what their responsibilities are through clear job descriptions and standards of performance. They need to how they well they are doing via ongoing informal and formal feedback through one-on-one regular meetings with their supervisor and a periodic formal evaluation. Once everyone knows the rules, they know how to function well in their roles.

Train your brains.
It is your responsibility to make sure your people have the training they need to do their jobs well. There is nothing more frustrating

than having a responsibility and lacking the knowledge or skills to do it. On the other hand, learning new things stimulates your mind and brings satisfaction. It keeps you from being bored, provides a sense of accomplishment, and avoids inordinately focusing on interpersonal relationships.

I was well-trained in medicine when I went to the mission field, but had no concept how little I knew about fulfilling my missionary role well. Looking back, what I found most satisfying was learning new things. During my time in Kenya, I learned about management, administration, governance, foundation grant writing, construction, project development, milking a cow, raising chickens, water containment, drip irrigation, running a greenhouse, operating a shortwave radio, starting a nursing school, writing computer programs, being a leader, snorkeling, computerizing a hospital, firing someone, building a hydroelectric system, running a meeting, making a movie, playing squash, being a tour guide, and the list goes on and on.

Stimulate your people with on-the-job training, in-house continuing education, and formal outside training opportunities. The work you are doing is too important not to train your employees.

Recognize people's accomplishments.
It is human nature to want our achievements recognized. Work hard to catch your people doing good things and compliment them. Pass on comments people share about their work by placing a comment box in your facility, doing a written feedback survey with your patients, or doing some sporadic oral interviews as patients leave. Recognize people for their years of service and personalize it the best you can. We recognize employees for each five years they serve with us on an escalating level of recognition. I write a note to each employee and we give each one a significant gift that grows in value at each anniversary. We have our staff members nominate and then vote on the "Staff Servant of the Year." We give merit bonuses to outstanding achievers.

Interestingly, the staff members pour their gratitude back to us to an embarrassing degree and have lots of fun doing it. On Boss' Day one year, the theme was "Don't get used to it!" The staff members spoiled Dr. Rudd and me all day by chauffeuring us to work in a Cadillac, serving us tea and crumpets, and giving us massages. They even created and wrote articles expressing their gratitude and printed them on the front and back pages of a newspaper that they gave to us to read with our morning slippers and cups of coffee at our desks. Each department also created their own "event" to pamper us. But at each event throughout the day, they reminded us, "Don't get used to it." It was certainly a memorable day!

Create an atmosphere of inordinate gratitude and recognition to pour fragrant oil on your team. Have a goat roast or some other sort of feast, organize contests, and get your staff involved in recognizing each other's accomplishments.

Communicate to connect.
On a quarterly basis, I set aside time during our regular chapel time to hold a "town meeting" to give the staff an overview of what is going on and assess where we are as an organization. I relate facts, but brag on individual and departmental accomplishments. I work hard to give them the big picture and show how their individual parts are making a difference while mixing it with humor and some stories. Informally, this happens all the time through sharing prayer requests, monthly reports, and notes from members, as well as having individuals come and share how CMDA impacted their lives, as well as through our publications which we internally circulate.

Good communication is the grease in the wheels of your organization that helps you from wearing out your bearings. These meetings are recorded and sent to staff members not in attendance. Also look for formal and informal ways for your staff to communicate with you and other leaders in your organization. People are less likely to get frustrated when they have channels to vent their concerns, and you won't get blindsided by a blowup when you didn't even know there was a problem.

Schedule some laughter.
Make memories together by scheduling some fun times. Don't worry; you don't have to think up what to do. Just set a small group of your most imaginative staff loose with a date and a budget, and tell them to be as creative as possible. You are looking for unpredictable fun and laughter wrapped around some meaningful moments.

Our Christmas party one year lasted four hours. We dismissed work early and the party committee wowed us. We laughed, shed a few tears, and had our hearts moved. Everyone was asked to come to the party dressed in a Bethlehem costume. To make it easy, we borrowed costumes from a local church for those who didn't have time to create one. We had a random ornament exchange to pick our prayer partner for the year, made paper figures to put in the manger displays that served as our table centerpieces, played Christmas story trivia with prizes (An extra half day of vacation is a wonderful motivator!), had a progressive Christmas play with members of the audience being picked to perform, enjoyed great food, listened to good music, received a Christmas message, and much more. We still talk about it and share pictures on our staff website. That event and other fun times throughout the year coat our relationships with Teflon.

Be predictably unpredictable.
Everyone likes a pleasant surprise. You have to be more creative when you have patients to take care of, but look for ways to show your staff you care. One Thursday, we invited our staff to come to the lobby, bring a bowl, and get some popcorn. Once a month after chapel, we celebrate the month's birthdays with homemade desserts served in the kitchen. One Christmas, our finances did not allow us to give a large bonus, so we gave each staff member an extra day of vacation just before the regular holidays.

We have our traditions, but we also work hard at being unpredictable so staff members don't get bored or see something as an entitlement. Some of this unpredictability focuses on individual staff members, just a department, or even the whole group. It might be a lunch out, a card when someone is ill, flowers after the death of a loved one, or a gag gift.

Lest you think all we do is play, I should mention that our staff members are very high performers. Pouring oil in the gears takes some time and a little bit of money, but it avoids costly repairs or unfixable breakdowns. When combined with seeing and dealing with interpersonal problems early and a high expectation that people are expected to love one another, it leads to great achievements. Best of all, people are having fun getting there! How can you put some oil in the gears?

CHAPTER 25
TO CATCH A THIEF

Do you remember the suavely handsome Cary Grant and the soon-to-be princess Grace Kelley in the Oscar winning movie *To Catch a Thief*? A reformed jewel thief is suspected of returning to his former occupation and has to ferret out the real culprit in order to prove his innocence. The cat burglar has to be wily to catch the mouse that is eating other people's cheese. I didn't know when I headed overseas as a medical missionary that catching thieves would also be part of my job description.

Many places in the world are full of corruption—embezzlement, theft, graft, and bribery. The problem is compounded by poverty and family obligations. Family members with jobs are expected to help with school fees. Men are often under huge pressure to acquire a dowry before getting married. In other places, parents may need to amass significant wealth to pay both a dowry and wedding costs. These pressures can be overwhelming, even for Christians, and sometimes people succumb.

Unfortunately, mission institutions and leaders are not exempt from dealing with these issues. I remember some days feeling more like a policeman than a missionary as I battled the numerous ways staff, patients, and outsiders attempted to steal from our hospital and clinics.

- Sheets, blankets, and pillows were thrown over the fence to friends and relatives or hidden under clothes as people went home.
- People snuck out of the hospital without paying their bills.
- A clerk replaced the carbon paper in the receipt book with a piece of cardboard. Later he put a piece of paper and carbon

paper over the duplicate receipt and wrote in a lesser amount and then pocketed the difference. Over time he stole a huge amount of money.
- Armed robbers broke into the hospital one night, broke down the business office door, and stole the hospital's cash.
- A cook took a large bag of beans and hid it in his home.
- Medical equipment and medicines were stolen by staff so they could open their own "clinics" in the community. Most of them had little medical education.
- Empty antibiotic bottles were taken, filled with aspirin or other cheap medicines, and sold as antibiotics.
- Used syringes and empty vials were taken, filled with water, and used by "private practitioners" to inject patients.
- Medicine dispensers would give the patients half or none of their medicine doses and put the pills in their own pockets.

I could go on and on, but here is the point. As good stewards, we have the duty to stem the tide of pilfering and larceny to ensure we have the resources to treat patients and avoid people in the community being hurt by charlatans. Here are a few principles I learned that might be helpful to you.

Hire the Right People for the Right Jobs
I finally realized that I was corrupting good Christian men if I asked them to handle money. Women had fewer pressures and were more resistant to embezzlement and theft. So I made a policy that only women could work in the business office if at all possible. If not, we picked men who did not have financial pressures, were strong Christians, and had a long record of honesty in other places.

Decrease Temptation
If items could not be sold or used easily, the temptation to steal them decreased. We imprinted our logo on sheets, towels, drapes, and every other thing made of wood or cloth. We engraved it on metal objects. We threw empty pill bottles, vials, and syringes into the "placenta pit"—a deep hole in the ground full of placentas, body parts removed during surgery, and other biological waste that no one was going to get near. We stored patients' street clothes and gave them hospital clothes clearly identifying them as patients so it was almost impossible to go AWOPYB—Absent without Paying Your Bill.

Make it Hard to Steal
We were one of the first mission hospitals to computerize in the late 1980s. Not only did computers prevent math errors in calculating patient bills, but they kept medicine/supply costs updated and provided valuable management information. They also made it very difficult to falsify receipts. We had a high fence around the hospital and guards at our gates. Bags and containers that visitors carried in were stored at the visitors' entrance or inspected upon going in and out. We limited access to central supply, warehouses, the laundry, and other places where valuable equipment, supplies, and medicines were stored.

Accountability
We instituted inventory systems and held people accountable for the things they were entrusted with. We put inventory numbers on equipment and checked that the items were present. We did spot checks to make sure medicines and supplies requisitioned were used as intended. We had an outside audit of the hospital's funds. We posted signs asking patients to inform senior management if their receipts or bills were inaccurate. We handled and counted money with at least two people.

Rewards and Recognition
We taught and inspired honesty and rewarded departments and individuals who excelled in their internal audits and prevented theft. This recruited staff to work with us to prevent theft, as well as recognized top performers.

Consequences
The employees learned by experience that they would simply be fired if they were caught stealing. That led to the theory you could steal as much as possible, and just go home and enjoy your ill-gotten gains if you were caught. To reverse this, we adopted the philosophy used by retail stores and put up signs saying "Shoplifters Will Be Prosecuted." We informed our staff and the public that they would be arrested and prosecuted if they were caught stealing.

And it wasn't just a threat; we actually followed through on it when theft was detected. The first case was a head clerk in the business office who was falsifying receipts. His scheme was exposed when a patient brought back a receipt after partial payment of a bill and it did not match the carbon copy in the receipt book. Our investigation revealed he had stolen the equivalent of fifteen years' worth of salary and probably more than that. We reported it to the police and they arrested him. The case dragged on for almost a year.

Finally he was sentenced to one month in prison for each of the fifteen counts of theft we could get patients to register complaints about. I thought it should have been much more, but it still had the desired effect. It deterred theft.

Consistency
Systems with checks and balance are useless if you aren't consistent in ensuring they continue to operate. You also have to lay out the consequences for mistakes or intentional theft and then take action when these situations occur.

Persistence
People will continually think up new ways to line their pockets. The necessity and desperation they feel is the mother of invention. You have to continually adapt to changing threats.

Sometimes things will not go well. The cook who stole was caught red handed by the police with our marked burlap bag full of beans in his house and was arrested. But we had a corrupt judicial system. A family member bribed the judge who not only declared him innocent but demanded that we hire him back to his former position. Despite that setback, we continued to persist by appealing his case and following through on all of our policies and procedures.

Get Everyone Involved
You don't want it to appear as though the missionaries are the only ones involved in security. Both national and missionary leadership must present a united front. Security issues should be discussed by management staff members and they must be involved in setting up the system and enforcing it.

Exhibit Grace and Forgiveness
You may ask, "But what will people think of you as a Christian and missionary? Won't you hurt your efforts in evangelism and disciple-

ship?" The Bible teaches we must love the sinner but punish the sin if we are in a place of authority.

I remember traveling down the rough dirt road to Tenwek on a return trip from a business meeting. Walking down that same road was the young man we had prosecuted for stealing who was in prison for fifteen months. As he served his time in a distant facility, I was unable to visit him but prayed for him regularly. I stopped, picked him up, and asked how he was doing. I told him I was very sorry for the effect his imprisonment had on him and his family, but we couldn't let a crime go unreported.

He turned to me and said, "Dr. Stevens, I want to thank you for putting me in prison." I'm sure my jaw must have fallen open.

He went on, "I was in despair when I was first put in my cell. I thought about killing myself. I had disgraced myself and my family. My wife was pregnant. But God brought me to a local pastor who volunteered as a chaplain. I knew about Christ and could even talk the language of a Christian, but I realized I needed Christ as my Savior and Lord when I hit bottom in that prison. The chaplain led me to Christ and I accepted Him into my life on my knees in that cell.

"Then I grew in Christ. I had lots of time to study His word! Within a month or two, I was sharing the gospel regularly with other prisoners and became the chaplain's unofficial assistant. I probably never would have come to Christ if I hadn't gone to prison!"

I found out he couldn't find a job because of his prison record, so I hired him back to work at the hospital. Of course, I didn't put him back in the business office. He joyfully mowed lawns and I would find him in the chapel sharing his testimony with patients during his tea break.

Show love and, when appropriate, grace. God can use difficult circumstances to accomplish His plans. Maybe you don't have security problems where you work. If so, praise the Lord and pray for those who do. If you do, these principles served me well. I hope they do the same for you.

PART 7
MISSIONAL SITUATIONS

CHAPTER 26
SPIRITUAL MINISTRY IN MEDICAL MISSIONS

We've waded through learning how to develop a strategic plan and other important topics for your mission. Hard work, isn't it? Now let's deal with the most important issue in your medical mission outreach—how do you reach people with the gospel?

Realize that the devil will do everything possible to keep you from making this goal your most important priority. His favorite weapon is unlimited medical needs and limited personnel, resources, and funding. With all you have to do, how can you focus your time and energy on this area? Relax! As a physician, you really have only two or three responsibilities, and I will cover each one of them in detail.

Everyone's situation is different, so I'm going to focus on principles with a few examples and ideas that worked for us in Kenya. As you may know, Kenya is a Christian country and is open to the gospel, which made evangelism and discipleship easier. Your place of service is likely to be different, but the principles will work no matter where you are located. The application will change with every situation.

Your first major responsibility is making sure spiritual ministry is happening. You can't focus much of your own time in doing it, but you need someone totally focused on making it happen. When I led World Medical Mission, I toured various mission hospitals and always asked about spiritual ministry. I remember one evangelical hospital had a pastor come to visit patients two half-days a week. It was a large hospital with 200 beds and many staff, but the administration didn't think spiritual ministry was as important as having nurses, doctors, and lab technicians.

If spiritual ministry is the most important thing, then that department should be better staffed than any area of your ministry. Sooner or later, every patient you treat is going to die. You are just putting off the inevitable with medicine and treatment. Only when they are introduced to Christ as their Savior can they live forever.

You should carefully pick your head chaplain.
They should be an "A" employee who cannot only do the job better than you, but is also a visionary and implementer. Pay this person well, at least at the level of other senior staff. It will be money well invested. This person should at least have a Bible college level education.

Give stature to the head chaplain's position.
This chaplain should be a member of your senior staff, involved in strategic planning, and a part of your routine management meetings to determine how the hospital will function. You and all your staff need someone who is always thinking, "How will this decision impact our spiritual ministry?"

Train your chaplains.
You can be a great pastor and a very poor chaplain. The roles are completely different. At the minimum, hire people who have a passion for sharing the gospel and have done so in their daily lives. Then send them for specific chaplaincy training. I'm not talking about a seminary degree, though that may be helpful. I'm talking about learning how to be a chaplain from really good chaplains. Where do you find someone like that? Visit *www.tenwek.com* to learn about the L. Nelson Bell Chaplaincy Training School led by Dr. David Kilel, the head chaplain at Tenwek. It offers two-month courses of varied lengths using both lecture and hands-on application in the hospital.

David is one of the best one-on-one soul winners I've ever met and a terrific chaplain. Each year at Tenwek, around 3,000 patients and their families make spiritual decisions. Learning from an effective program will give your chaplains the tools, ideas, and networks needed to be effective. The friends they make during training will be a great support group to encourage their work.

By the way, how would you like to be the only doctor in a 200-bed hospital? You couldn't do a very good job. Over time, you would likely burn out with the unending night calls and emergencies. Yet, we often ask a single chaplain to provide routine and emergency services for a facility that size. Hire enough chaplains to do the work.

Make spiritual ministry an integral part of the hospital's activities.
At Tenwek, we had chapel every morning at 10 a.m. The chapel stood right in the center of the hospital. Doctors on rounds were expected to stop seeing patients unless it was an emergency, so I would make myself scarce by reading x-rays or doing a procedure during this time. Why? If patients saw me making rounds, they didn't go to chapel because they were worried they would miss the doctor. When the chapel bell rang, I would say to the patients in the ward, "I encourage you to go to the chapel service. I will be back to finish rounds at 10:30."

For those who couldn't attend chapel, we held services in their area—maternity, isolation, and outpatients—at the same time. We also had an ongoing ministry to outpatients since people came and went all day. A TV played the "Jesus video" or other outreach materials in each waiting area. The only downfall being that patients were often so intent on watching the film they didn't hear their name called to go into the exam room!

I can say much more about your hospital's spiritual outreach, but let me interject to focus on your second main responsibility. You are responsible for setting the priority of the spiritual ministry by example. In other words, you need to be doing evangelism. Yes, I know that you don't have time to witness to every patient, but you need to look for those God impresses on you to share the gospel. Speak in chapel every once in a while. Pray before surgery. Write spiritual consults for patients you see need a chaplain. Hold a Bible study in your home with some of your senior staff. You will get your greatest satisfaction not from a dramatic lifesaving emergency C-section but from leading someone to the Lord!

Let me give you some other tips.

- Set up a regular time to meet with the head chaplain to discuss the spiritual ministry and how to improve it. This sends a powerful message and lets you nurture this key staff member.

- Budget for spiritual ministry resources such as tracts, videos, and discipleship materials.
- Help your chaplain develop a follow-up system with new converts to get them established in a local church. We found that others in the family came to Christ if a chaplain did a follow-up visit with new converts. Your medical ministry can fuel church growth and new church planting.
- Have your chaplains train your hospital staff to do outreach to patients. Everyone should be part of the spiritual outreach team.
- Encourage staff to minister on the wards in the evenings and on weekends by organizing singing groups, sharing testimony, or preaching.
- Collect the names and contact information of those who make decisions.
- Get your short-term volunteers involved in spiritual ministry by speaking in chapel or sharing their faith with patients via a translator. Make sure they get out into the community for services. It will be the highlight of their stay.
- Have the chaplain minister to your staff as well through counseling, regular services, Bible study groups, and outreach teams.
- Encourage hospital staff to focus on an outside ministry. About 30 staff members from Tenwek participate in a medical missions trip each October to a distant underserved area of the country. They offer medical services, but about a third of the team does a building project and another third does evangelism in the villages. While the hospital contributes a token amount, the involved staff and other team members cover the major cost of the trip.
- Sponsor an outside speaker for a special week of services for your staff each year.
- Recognize your chaplains' hard work at an annual staff party at Christmas or another occasion.
- Make sure your chaplains are growing and developing personally and professionally by sending them to conferences, giving them study helps, purchasing training videos or books, etc.

When we talked about strategic planning, we talked about goal setting. Make sure to measure and set individual goals for your chaplains. I remember David Kilel coming back to minister for a week during break from his seminary training. When I greeted him and asked how he was doing, he shared he had prayed and felt the Lord was going to give him the opportunity to win 50 patients to the Lord that week. With joy on his face, he pulled out a book from his pocket and showed me 64 names of those who came to Christ. What gets measured gets done, so there should be concrete goals measuring both efforts and results in spiritual ministry.

What if you are in a creative access country or other harder to reach areas? You still need to be involved in personal outreach and make sure you have the right people focused on spiritual outreach in your ministry.

When I led a medical relief team into Mogadishu in the midst of famine, war, and dire medical needs, we were swamped with patients. We would see 500 patients or more a day. We couldn't stand up and preach or even hand out tracts. If we did, someone in this radical Muslim country would put a live grenade in our pockets. We prayed and discussed before finally realizing our primary ministry focus needed to be the 30 or more Somalis working with our team as translators, nurses, guards, etc. The one time when we all got together when we talked was to pack pill packets for the next day. With lots of prayer, we asked them to bring their Korans when we all got together to pack pills for the next day. During the next week or two, we asked them to tell us everything about being a Muslim as we packed pills. We then asked if we could bring our Bibles to tell them about what we believed as Christians. Many came to Christ, and some became active in evangelism to their friends and began Bible studies where they lived. I remember one man led more than 100 individuals to Christ, and he asked me to bring Bibles in for each of them. He became our "chaplain."

We followed the two main principles. We did outreach ourselves and then identified a key national to head up our spiritual ministry on a full-time basis. With intention, prayer, and focus, you can have a vibrant spiritual ministry through your healthcare outreach. If you already have an outreach, isn't it time to focus your efforts on making it better? "Seek ye first the kingdom of God" and all the medical and surgical duties you have to handle "will be added unto you."

CHAPTER 27
MEDICAL MISSIONS STAT!

Medical missionaries increasingly find themselves in proximity of or are asked to respond to natural and man-made disasters from tsunamis to earthquakes, famines to civil wars, epidemics to ethnic cleansings. If you haven't confronted any of these yet, just wait. Sooner or later you probably will.

I have a bit of experience in these areas. For two and a half years, I led medical relief teams for Samaritan's Purse into Bosnia, Somalia, Sudan, and Rwanda, so I am aware of the issues involved. Perhaps some of my reflections and considerations might be helpful to you one day when you face "medical missions STAT!"

If the catastrophe occurs around your place of service, it is obvious that providing medical relief is necessary. Your spectrum of disease will change, your volume of work will significantly increase, and you will face many logistical problems. But one dilemma you won't face is trying to decide whether or not you will be involved. You will be. But what if the catastrophe is in another section of your country or in a nearby country? Should you get involved?

Historically, medical missionaries have ventured to the most dangerous and difficult places; though, secular groups have increasingly taken the lead as they have been favored with funding from both individuals and secular governments. Let's look at the benefits of providing emergency medical relief. First, emergency medical personnel can gain access to countries or regions traditionally closed to missionaries, such as radical Muslim countries. When I led a medical team into Somalia, only about 300 Christians were estimated to be in Mogadishu with only a handful more in the entire country. Traditionally,

Christian organizations were not allowed in the country, but as the government had collapsed due to a civil war and famine, there was no government enforcement. Military and UN intervention provided a small window of relative stability where Christian relief organizations and missionaries could have an impact.

Secondly, in the midst of tragedy, people normally resistant to the gospel may be much more open to it. When they see Christian charity, they wonder what motivates such risky love to be manifested. They are attracted to our Lord through love and service.

Third, the Bible tells us to have mercy on those suffering.

- "Mercy to the needy is a loan to God, and God pays back those loans in full" (Proverbs 19:17, MSG).
- "God told Moses, 'I'm in charge of mercy. I'm in charge of compassion.' Compassion doesn't originate in our bleeding hearts or moral sweat, but in God's mercy" (Romans 9:15, MSG).
- "Real wisdom, God's wisdom, begins with a holy life and is characterized by getting along with others. It is gentle and reasonable, overflowing with mercy and blessings..." (James 3:17, MSG).

There are many more practical reasons to consider doing relief as well.

- Funding – It is often much easier to fund this type of outreach due to media attention. At least for a while, money will pour in to help people in need.
- Transport – Parastatal and government organizations may provide free transport. When I was doing relief work, often the UN or various government military organizations were willing to take us to needy areas and transport supplies and equipment. In Sudan, we were trying to halt the spread of an epidemic of relapsing fever. The UN let us fill most of a C-130 transport plane with tents, a large boat, motors, food, supplies, and medical equipment, and then they dropped us off at a remote dirt strip next to a river leading to the epicenter of the epidemic.
- Church Expansion – Our presence was a great help in expand-

ing the local church in that animistic area. It grew by leaps and bounds during the next nine months.
- Recruitment – Surprisingly, It Is easier to recruit at least short-term personnel for emergency situations. Somalia was in terrible turmoil when I arrived to survey the situation in 1992. I wondered if I could find anyone willing to go with our teams. We had medical personnel come out of the woodwork, many with significant experience in short- and long-term missions, and others who were neophytes, but God had moved in their hearts. We had to turn people down for lack of room.

There is also the ancillary benefit of being salt and light to the military and other relief organizations involved in the work. In Mogadishu, we had military healthcare personnel arrive in droves to participate in our weekly church services and assist in our work on their days off. They were not allowed to use military medicines and supplies to help the local people, but they had a great desire to relieve the suffering they saw each day. When they came as volunteers, they also brought all their security people with them which made our job safer and more organized. On Sundays, we made homemade cookies and other foods to give them a touch of home in a country far away. Having lots of single females on our team was an attraction as well! A good number of soldiers came to Christ and others grew in their faith because of our presence.

Another aspect to consider is the medical and cultural experience of long-term missionaries and their language knowledge. They are invaluable in an emergency. They have learned to adapt and "make-do" in challenging situations. They know the illnesses and cost-effective therapies that work in their region of the world. They may know where to get supplies, food, and other resources from local sources much cheaper than bringing them long distances.

Of course, the publicity the home mission organization gets as they respond to urgent needs may be widely disseminated by the media, often resulting in increasing the number of individuals, foundations, and even government organizations providing support for additional long-term endeavors.

But relief work has its downside as well. How will your present ministry continue to function while you're involved in this added outreach? Relief work requires a rapid, almost instantaneous response and is very costly. In Mogadishu, it cost $400 per day to rent just one vehicle, and we needed a number of them to transport our team to feeding centers and other ministry sites. In the early days we had to transport all of our medicine, food, supplies, and even water by air from Nairobi. Relief work is never self-supporting by patient fees. In most situations, even minimal fees can't be charged.

In civil wars or other violent situations, relief can be dangerous. In Somalia, we had ten guards carrying machine guns at our house compound and others in every vehicle leaving through the gate. Without those guards, we would have been robbed and possibly shot and killed. In Sudan, our team did not have guards and we were kidnapped and held hostage for a couple of days. Another time, we had to do an emergency evacuation as a tribal conflict resulted in a raid of the village where we were working, and many villagers were killed. In Rwanda, the killing teams washed the blood off their machetes in the hospital compound where we worked. There was no direct threat to the team, but continual danger exists in lawless situations.

One of the goals in missions is long-term sustainable development with ultimate nationalization and a long-term partnership with an indigenous church. It is difficult to set up and maintain infrastructures long-term in emergencies. You have to make extraordinary efforts to work with the local church if there is one, even though it is often in disarray due to the catastrophe. The people of the church are trying to survive just like everyone else.

I falsely imagined that all the relief organizations would have a sense of camaraderie and would work together. I was surprised to find that most agencies are uncooperative and territorial. An agency's existence is dependent on the press coverage it receives because the publicity brings in donations and grants to fund the group. There is competition for the most public and worthy work sites and sometimes even a deliberate sabotaging of the work of Christian groups. In Sudan, a well-known international medical group was setup down the river, and they tried to get us thrown out of the country by complaining to the UN because we were "proselytizing" by showing the "Jesus Film." In reality, they could have easily gotten extra funding and publicity if they were involved in addressing the epidemic of relapsing fever where we were—at the epicenter.

The Lords of Poverty is a book that scathingly addresses this and other issues of secular relief organizations that run from one disaster to another following the money with little thought to proper disengagement or turning the work into long-term development. When press coverage and funding dries up, these groups often leave immediately with no thought of the consequences to the local people.

In the above instance, the UN told us that we would no longer be allowed to use its flights to ferry personnel and supplies into the country unless we stopped witnessing. At that time, all flights other than UN flights were being shot down by the government air force. This action would have driven us out of Sudan. I had to show the UN workers a copy of their own charter which says everyone has a right to practice their own religious beliefs as well as to propagate these beliefs. This is only one example of how you may encounter and deal with organizations with considerable antagonism toward Christian organizations.

Of course, the hardest part of emergency medical relief is logistics. You are working in chaos without normal communication, transportation, housing, or supply systems; yet you have to move, lodge, feed, and find clean water, in addition to having the medical and other supplies available that you need to make a difference. You must be able to communicate. Before satellite phones, shortwave and VHF radio networks worked from your base to mobile units. I still remember hunching under the parapet on our flat roof house in Mogadishu to avoid sniper fire as I tried to operate our satellite fax machine to send a message to the U.S. I felt like James Bond.

Because the situation is changing so rapidly, it is difficult to set budgets or project costs or impact. A relief team requires intense support from a well-run organization outside the disaster to perform and meet the challenges it faces, and still everyone must acknowledge that the effort may end at any time due to circumstances beyond their control.

Let's talk about the mechanics of "medical missions STAT." Once you make a decision to be involved in relief efforts, how do you start? The first step is a rapid assessment. One or preferably two experienced people need to go into the crisis situation. That is easier said than done since the usual avenues of transportation, housing, security, communication, and food may no longer exist. We would usually send two people in, one with extensive medical experience and one with logistical experience. Going in pairs helps with security and, as the saying goes, "Two heads are better than one." It also helps both people process and cope with the psychological trauma of the devastation and suffering they will face. It can be overwhelming. The assessment team needs to be as self-contained as possible. In this day and time, that would ideally include the following items.

Instant Communications
For example, a satellite phone for text and voice communications. This will allow more rapid reporting and marshaling of resources from outside the crisis zone, provide reassurance of safety on a regular basis, assist in coordination with other relief, government, or international organizations, and help prepare emergency evacuation plans in case of trauma or serious illness.

Self-Contained Living Resources
Without hotels, restaurants, places to buy supplies, etc., it is a good idea to take a sleeping bag, concentrated food supplies, emergency medicines, digital cameras to document the situation (your organization will want pictures to publicize the need), and a small computing device to store pictures, take notes, record expenses, etc. Travel as light as possible since the weight allowance on relief transport is limited and you may have to carry it all yourself for significant distances on the ground.

Lots of Money
Dollars or other hard currency in both large and small denominations is essential. Use a money belt, but separate funds out into different locations. Know that if you take more than $10,000 out of the states, you must declare it to customs. (A "helpful" customs official at John F. Kennedy International Airport reminded me of that when I was carrying a large amount of cash from the U.S. to Somalia to fund our team!) Why "lots?" Because you may have to rent vehicles, planes, or other modes of transport to get there. You may need to secure lodging for

the team that will follow, buy or rent vehicles, hire security, purchase supplies, or even "buy" yourself out of a difficult situation. There are no credit card services in these situations and the price of the few remaining forces will escalate rapidly.

Health
All relief workers should be highly immunized. You don't know what diseases you will run into. Also carry one or more ways to decontaminate water. I used to carry iodine tablets as well as a small filtration system. Take a supply of medicines to cover likely contingencies, and I often carried a small surgical kit and suture.

Other
Take various forms of identification. Of course, you need your passport and a visa if required, but also take an organizational I.D. card. I did this in a form that I could hang around my neck and that could be seen from a distance. Another option is a jacket or t-shirt that identifies you. This is especially important in war situations but also is useful for pictures. It clearly identifies you in public relation shots. I also often carried "press" identification (even if it was actually Samaritan's Purse "press" tags). Press tags are easily recognized and honored in difficult situations. Letters of introduction from the UN or other organizations are helpful, and of course carry plenty of business cards for dealing with government or other officials.

The assessment team's job is to answer questions like:

- Who? – What variety of personnel is needed based on the type of needs? Do we need to do surgery for trauma, deal with a cholera epidemic, or initiate an immunization campaign?
- What Relief Work? – How can the most good for the most people be done in the shortest time with our available resources? What needs can our group meet that aren't better met by others? What should our relief and spiritual strategies be?
- Where? – Where should we base the team and where do we focus our work? Where is safe enough to work but dangerous enough that we are needed? Where can we sustain the team but still meet significant needs?
- How? – Logistics are the most difficult nut to crack. How are we going to house our relief team, feed them, provide water

for them, transport them, and keep them safe?
- With Whom? – Who do we need to liaison and cooperate with in this effort? Do we need to liaison with the UN, Red Cross, military, a rebel group, or other entities?

As assessment is taking place, several resources need to be organized back on the home front.

- Money – Funds need to be raised through appeals, the media, and your website with frequent visual, audio, and written reports describing the needs and how the donor funds will be used. It is helpful if the assessment team can digitally send pictures over the satellite phone.
- Personnel – Personnel need to be recruited. I used to make a short list of experienced people and personally contact them to ask them to go. It is almost mandatory to cover these volunteers' expenses and even pay a small stipend for incidentals, especially to those who stay a significant amount of time.
- Supplies and Equipment – You will need to obtain supplies, medicines, and equipment. Get these as close to the service site as possible to avoid costly transportation costs. When we were "camping" in Sudan, we bought boats, motors, generators, tents, food, and other items in Nairobi. You may need to set up a forward base at this supply point with a logistician that handles purchasing, houses relief workers going in and out of the work area, arranges transport, etc.

The next step is to lead the team to the location. Those on the assessment team either lead or go with the team. We often left the logistician in the area needing relief since the organization on the ground took more time than the medical assessment. Then the medical leader went back and brought the team to the location.

There will be a great deal of decisions to be made and much organization to do on the ground. Local national staff will need to be hired, routines developed, work sites established, and much more. Spiritual ministry will have to be developed which will differ significantly in different countries and situations. In Somalia, our target population was our forty Somali staff members. A quarter of these workers came to Christ and became vibrant witnesses bringing others to Christ too.

If you are providing relief for an extended period of time in a difficult situation, it is very stressful on your team members. It is wise to rotate them out for rest and restoration periodically. We used to do six weeks in-country and two weeks out for long-term staff. We had a core of these staff members and then brought in others for a few weeks to a month to supplement their efforts.

As the team leader, I was in-country for an extended period of time. Once the team was on the ground, I then went back and forth to the forward base and the U.S. for recruiting. There were many dealings with officials, reporting, taking the video team in, and heading many other activities. We had a ministry site leader who took over the day-to-day duties.

In a relief situation, the situation changes from day-to-day, but over time one of two things will happen. The security situation could get so bad in a war or other conflict situation and you will have to pull your team out, often on very short notice. A quick exit plan is an important part of your contingency planning.

The other thing that could happen is that the acute relief needs are met and you will need to disengage. This may be transforming your work into long-term medical or development outreach yourself or turning your efforts over to nationals. It is important if you do the latter to continue to provide support and finances until they can be self-sustaining.

Most of all, this type of work needs lots of prayer support. It is not easy; it is dangerous and unpredictable. But God does His best work in crisis situations, that is His specialty. You will learn to depend on Him in new ways and see His hand more clearly. That alone is worth the risk of "medical missions STAT!" And it's what He calls you to do.

CHAPTER 28
PERFECTING YOUR PRAYER LETTER

I need to confess something to you that I'm ashamed to admit. I only hope you can handle the truth! I don't read all the missionary prayer letters I receive. Okay. There. I've said it.

Many are so poorly written that I skim them or just read the captions under the pictures. Sometimes the pictures are so poor that I can't bear to even do that. In fact, today I'm reading a lower percentage of the letters I receive than ever before because I'm getting more and more letters with the advent of e-mail service in remote missionary sites.

How can you perfect your prayer letter? How can you build affinity (a natural liking for or inclination towards somebody) with this important missionary tool? It can be done. In fact, I have a few missionary friends whose prayer letters I always look forward to getting. I read every word they write. What are they doing that you should do? Here is what I've learned that you need to do.

Know Them
Who gets your letter? What are they interested in? How can you build bridges from where they are to where you want to take them? Remember you have to start from where people exist in their experiences, attitudes, and knowledge. It can be difficult when you are corresponding with a long list of individuals, but ask, "What do they have in common in these areas?" Mentally construct a composite individual you are writing your prayer letter to, and write to that person.

Grab Them
If you say, "I was lost, night was falling and the lions were beginning

to roar," you will instantly grab the reader's attention and pull them in. Or you may share a quandary about a beggar child you met in an urban environment and begin, "How do you tell a starving child about Jesus?" I wrote a prayer letter when I was on the field which began, "I looked in every medical textbook I had, but there was nothing written about how to treat a hippo bite!" Get the idea? You want to grab the reader's attention and capture them for, as Paul Harvey says, "the rest of the story." The first paragraph, the lead to the letter, is critically important.

Theme It

What is the key point you want to get across? You should want to inspire, teach, convict, or give a new glimpse of God much more than just inform. You need to include your theme statement within the first two or three paragraphs. I still remember a letter I received from a missionary doctor more than ten years ago. His theme was "God is looking for 'peculiar' people." His point was looking for people who are courageous, adaptable, and cut from a different cloth.

Use the examples below for a few ideas to theme your letter.
- "No matter how dangerous the situation, God is there to see you through." The theme is trust in God.
- "First Christ met people at their point of need, ministered to them, and then introduced them to His father." We must first meet physical needs to earn the right to share the gospel.
- "It is your faithful prayers that see me through seemingly insurmountable challenges." The importance of prayer.

Get the idea? Answer the question, "What is the key message I want them to remember?" Most everything in the letter should support that key message.

Prove It

Use stories to punch your theme home. Tell about the beggar on the street, the unusual case, the trial, the danger, or whatever will prove your point. I wrote an article for our mission magazine that got rave reviews. The theme was God could sustain you through difficult times. I wrote a log of a very difficult and busy day in the hospital in a progress note style. I made my point as I described difficult cases, long hours, lack of tools, etc.

You don't have to limit yourself to stories. Compare and contrast from what people know to what you are telling them. What is something like or how does it differ? Simply telling people that your hospital serves 300,000 people does not have nearly as much impact as saying, "Can you imagine a city like Lexington, Kentucky, or Newark, New Jersey, only having a 125-bed hospital and three doctors to serve the entire city?" If you serve in a remote area, you could say, "Imagine driving from Washington, D.C. to Philadelphia, Pennsylvania, on a rutted, mud-holed dirt road with no gas stations, no restaurants, and no off ramps."

Use analogies to compare two things similar in some respects while helping to explain something by starting from a point people already understand. One of the favorite interviewees after a plane tragedy years ago was a stewardess. She said on national TV, "Maintenance on this airline is so poor they may as well be holding the planes together with duct tape." There was not one piece of duct tape used in maintenance, but her analogy made her point. People had done makeshift and unstable repairs.

Make sure to share your emotions and feelings, not just the facts. People want to know the impact the story, statistic, or situation had on you. For example, if you were doing a challenging case without the right instruments you could say, "I was scared but I was the patient's only hope, even if I did not have the instrument I needed to control the bleeding. My soul cried out, 'God… help me.'"

Picture It
A picture may be worth a thousand words, but it is much more effective if it goes along with your story. Get in the habit of carrying your camera. (After a few years on the field, I know it is easy to not bother.) Take the time to get a picture to illustrate your story or point; for goodness sake, make sure you are in the picture. The best picture of the accident you had when your car slid off the road into the ditch is not a picture of the car lying on its side. Instead, the best picture is the one with you and a dozen passersby trying to right it. Hand your camera to someone else and get in the picture.

Here are some other picture tips:
- Get close. In your prayer letter, the pictures will be small.

- Always use fill flash, especially if you work in a country with dark skinned people. The flash will fill in the shadows and dark parts.
- Go digital and then crop, improve the contrast, lighting, etc. in a photo editing program.
- Caption the picture if it needs it for understanding.
- Do not use bad pictures. If the picture didn't turn out well, didn't print well, or has other problems, don't use it except in extraordinary situations. (It is okay to use a bad picture with this type caption: "Here is the picture when the rhino was chasing me. It is a little blurry, but you can understand why my wife Jody's hand wasn't so steady!") If you do not have a picture, describe the scene in detail (smells, sounds, sights) with your words.

Make Them Laugh
The best humor is when you make fun of yourself. The mistake you made in language school, the day your pants fell down during surgery (It happened to me!), or the funny picture of your two-year-old daughter who fell asleep on the dog will tickle people's funny bone.

Avoid Jargon
If you use medical terms, foreign words, or other phrases that people do not understand, explain them. Even some English phrases may not be understood if they are used differently in your country of call. People will scratch their heads if you say, "Jody went to the duka to get some napkins for the baby." Why not just say, "Jody went to the store to get diapers for the baby," unless there is some reason to take the time and space to explain these terms. Sometimes you do have reason to explain, such as, "The man fractured his skull with a 'rungut,' a highly polished and prized club carried by every man as a badge of manhood."

Share Specific Needs
Focus on your most important needs, but especially those needs that fit within your theme. "God does answer prayer. We are praying for you and need your prayers for these three important things." You may also mention needs for staff, work team members, funding, etc. The best needs to share are ones your readers can do something about through action or prayer.

Show the Product
What has their giving and praying accomplished? Whose health was restored? Whose heart was changed? Testimonies and stories are much more effective than blanket statements or statistics. "I just completed our annual report and was thrilled to find that more than 5,000 patients came to Christ last year." A powerful statement can be made even more powerful by following it with, "Those are not just numbers but individual lives transformed. Let me tell you about one of them."

Thank Them
Don't simply thank them the same way every time. Work hard to learn new ways to say thank you and remember you can't say thank you too many times or in too many ways.

Conclude It
Finish on your highest note. Go back to your theme and punch it home. Remember our three example lead sentences. You might conclude those letters with:
- "I've learned one thing. No matter how deep into the jungle of Africa I go, God is there taking care of me. He will take care of you in your 'jungles' too."
- "The Great Physician is an expert on treating hippo bites. I'm so thankful He stood by and guided me. Isn't it wonderful to know God is sufficient for all our needs?"
- "Starving children break my heart. I must reach out to nourish them, but I can't stop there. I have to remember their souls are starving as well, and they desperately need to know Christ. You may not see physical starvation like I do every day, but you see starving souls. Are you feeding them?"

I bet you are just as tired of humdrum prayer letters as I am. I know I am tired of reading travelogues ("I attended church in Longisa last Sunday, and then went to Nairobi on business for the hospital on Monday.") If your writing is not up to par, take out your last few letters and see how they measure up to these prayer letter principles. Then sit down and write your next prayer letter using these ideas. Let someone else critique it using these principles as guidelines. Incorporate their suggestions and send it out. A good letter is rewritten and polished a number of times.

Guess what? Before long, people will be devouring what you write and eagerly looking for your next correspondence. With practice, you can write the perfect prayer letter.

CHAPTER 29
RAISING BIG BUCKS

All of us need money for our medical ministries, and lots of it. Providing medical service is not cheap, even if your medical facility is self-supporting in its day-to-day operation. You still need a large fund available for the needy, as well as money for equipment, new buildings, training schools, and program help for community health/development evangelism. In fact, the list goes on and on. If you are in a mission that requires you to raise your own personal support, you know the challenge of going church to church. If you are supported by a denomination, they are unlikely to have the funds available to do all that needs to be done. So where do you raise the big bucks needed to ensure you can provide quality healthcare as well as have the opportunity to win people to Christ?

You may not realize it, but "funders" need you. Good projects and effective programs are not easily found. The job of these "funders" is to give away money. Foundations, trusts, and even some government programs are required to give away a set amount each year. The leaders of these groups have to show results to their boards or other overseeing bodies. They have to demonstrate they made a difference. You have an advantage with these groups, since you can movingly picture the need for your services in ways that many other outreaches cannot.

More and more, secular funding groups are looking with favor upon faith-based organizations (FBOs). The World Health Organization now admits that 30 to 70 percent of healthcare in Africa is provided by FBOs, and a recent Gallup Poll revealed that local people in 19 African countries put their greatest trust in religious organizations. Ample data is also available showing the ABC approach (A-for abstinence, B-for being faithful, and C-for consistent condom use) favored by FBOs is the most effective way to slow the AIDS epidemic.

So what keeps more major funders from finding you, and you from finding them? It is often due to a lack of knowledge of the other's existence or mutual interests. Commonly, medical missionaries lack the time, energy, or expertise to apply to the search. Often doctors are so overburdened by their patient responsibilities that they rarely have time to visit the capital to find funding organizations with offices in their service country or they lack internet access to search for assistance. Yet one of the keys to success in your ministry is the ability to find and organize financial and human resources. If you are a leader in your ministry, these are two of your most important tasks.

We were in the middle of a building project at Tenwek to provide operating rooms, seventy additional beds, and space for a small nursing school. But we had a problem. The project was costing more than anticipated and we were running out of funds.

My dad mentioned he knew a widow whose husband established a foundation focused on Africa. With no expertise but lots of determination, I sat down one Sunday afternoon and wrote her a three-page letter asking for money to build and fund the startup of the nursing school. I ran a draft for editing by the hospital CEO and then sent it off in the mail. Six weeks later, we got word the foundation gave us $150,000, which was a great deal of money in 1981. I remember thinking, "This is much easier than deputation! How many churches would I have to speak in to raise $150,000?"

During the next ten years, we raised more than $5 million to remodel and establish new buildings, staff housing, a hydroelectric plant, a sewage system, water treatment plant, and other capital projects. We funded our community outreaches, started a chaplaincy training school, bought equipment, and built visiting staff quarters. Let me share with you what I learned along the way.

Planning precedes the proposal. You need to be able to articulate your mission, vision, slogan, and values. You need to do an analysis and document the biggest issues you are facing now or will face in the future. Obtain as much hard data as you can so your proposal is not an opinion piece. Look for figures specific to your country to use as a backdrop, but add specific information on your service area. If necessary, conduct a survey of your target population. During a school break, we used schoolteachers to do a survey of 600 homes, and then worked with a U.S. school of public health to evaluate the data. You can also use hospital data. If you are not doing an annual report on your medical ministry, this is the time to start. It is needed to include with your proposal and also provides useful data to show problems needing to be addressed.

Prioritize your problems to address and develop a strategy to address them. How will you measure success? For example, if you want to decrease the incidence rate of morbidity and mortality from gastroenteritis, strategies may include teaching people how to use clean water, do oral rehydration, wash their hands, and build latrines. Success might be measured by a 40 percent increase in the number of homes with latrines, a 50 percent increase of mothers who know how to do ORS on a home survey, or a 60 percent increase in the number of water filtration systems you make and distribute. However, the most valuable data would be to demonstrate a decrease in gastroenteritis in the last two weeks on a home survey that correlates with decreased admissions for dehydration.

What funding will you need to hire staff, buy equipment, build buildings, or start programs to solve the problem you identified? Why is your organization especially suited to address this need? What are other organizations doing about this problem? Are you willing to network, work with them, or complement their efforts? Thinking through these areas is a key to acquiring the funding you need.

The next step is finding a funding organization. Start close to home. What groups are already funding you or other outreaches in your country? Who has offices in your country you could visit? Where are other mission hospitals getting outside funding? If you don't know, ask them. Are the groups you identify funding the types of needs you have? Some funding organizations want to fund programs while others may have more interest in bricks and mortar.

Ask someone to help you identify foundations in your own hometown or your staff's hometowns. Foundations love to help their native sons and daughters. When you are home on deputation, visit these groups and continue to ask who might be funders in your community. Don't forget to inquire about family foundations.

U.S. foundations are listed in the *Foundation Directory* published by the Foundation Center in New York. The directory is not cheap, but it is worth the cost. You can also access the online version at *http://fconline.foundationcenter.org/*. You can do multiple searches online to see what foundations are interested in healthcare or your country and give grants in the size you need. The directory lists the average size of the grant and some of the organizations they have supported. It also tells you how to apply and obtain more information.

For U.S. government programs, visit *www.fedmoney.com* and download the free Federal Money Retriever software. They also offer a free program called GrantGate.

Also check out American Schools and Hospitals Abroad, a USAID group that helps with capital development costs for institutions that "promote American values." They gave 50 percent of the funding needed for a number of large projects at Tenwek. They can be found online at *www.usaid.gov*.

There are also funding organizations in other countries. We received funding from EZE in Germany, a parastatal group that distributed millions of dollars of church taxes each year to developing countries. You often hear about organizations in Europe through word of mouth, but online searches can also be useful.

Develop a list of prospects to thoroughly investigate. The most important factor to consider is whether you know someone who works with or is on the board of the potential funding organization. No other factor correlates better with success. Also, be sure to use questions like the following to analyze and compare prospect groups in your database.

1. Has the foundation demonstrated a real commitment to funding the type of project you desire?
2. Does the foundation make grants to recipients in your geographical location?

3. Does the amount of money you are requesting fit within the foundation's grant range?
4. Does the foundation have any policy prohibiting grants for the type of support you are requesting?
5. Does the foundation like to make grants to cover the full cost of a project or only partial funding?
6. Does the foundation allow other foundations to share the cost of the project?
7. How long are typical grants for?
8. What is the time from application to decision?
9. Does the foundation have application deadlines or does it review proposals continuously?
10. Can you meet the foundation's reporting and managing requirements if a grant is awarded?
11. What kind of organizations does the foundation favor?
12. Can you meet the foundation's application requirements?

Your initial approach is often through a letter of inquiry. It should briefly describe who you are, the problem, the method you will use to address the issue, the cost, and the type and amount of support you are seeking over a period of time. I've found it useful to summarize as much as possible in the first paragraph similar to what a newspaper article does. This letter should be no longer than three pages. Don't forget to request application guidelines if needed.

When you get to the proposal, write it yourself. You know your situation best. Be clear and concise and give the facts. Stay within space guidelines and give the details requested. Spend sufficient time on your budget to think of everything—salaries, fringe benefits, consultant fees, utilities, equipment, supplies, travel, capital outlays, etc. Make sure to include the value of any contributions you or others are making in money or in kind. That should include the value of time, equipment, and building usage. You may want to value professional time at the salary level of your home country. Funding groups like to see your organization investing in the project.

A full list of current and recent sponsors can build your credibility. I always include or offer a copy of the organization's audited financial statements. Also let them know how you plan to continue the project or maintain the building after their funding is completed.

Most proposals should be ten to fifteen pages long, but you can include extra information—graphs, tables, references, etc.—in the appendix. Pictures to demonstrate the need and show your ministry's effectiveness can also be included in this section.

A week or two after your proposal is sent, send a follow-up letter or call to make sure your proposal arrived. Ask if there is any additional information they might find helpful. Invite them to visit or ask if you can visit them if it is a substantial request. Continue to follow-up on a regular basis until you get an answer.

If you get a rejection, don't give up. Foundations get more good proposals than they can fund. Ask the foundation how you can strengthen your proposal and whether they would let you submit your proposal again in their next funding period. Even if they say no, consider submitting another funding proposal to them within a year. Often you get two to three rejections before a foundation, especially one that does not know you, will say "yes."

If you get the grant, immediately write a letter of thanks. Get your project started, do what you said you would do, and do it on time. Your funding source will be impressed if you do, and they will be more likely to continue funding other projects you present. They like to stay in touch with good partners. I always tried to exceed our grantors expectations by doing extra things like sending pictures or acknowledging the foundation in print or other media. A gift of a memorable token of appreciation, such as a framed picture of the dedication with a citation or a before and after picture of someone who has been impacted by their grant, will make a great impression.

To sum it up, writing a proposal means selling yourself and your organization—don't be too humble. You need to convince them you are the best solution to solve the problem you are both concerned about. Always try to emphasize that your solution is innovative and will be replicable by other groups. Most of all, bathe the process in prayer. God knows your needs and can move in individual hearts and funding institutions. Go after the big bucks! It can revolutionize your health outreach.

PART 8
COMMUNITY PROJECTS

CHAPTER 30
TURBOCHARGING COMMUNITY HEALTH

A good community health program can save many more lives than curative services. I saw it happen as a young missionary doctor. When I arrived in Kenya, half of our admissions and half of our patient deaths were from preventable diseases. In those days, it was not unusual to do two to three cut downs a day on severely dehydrated children after multiple attempts to get IVs in them. We had an entire ward full of children with severe measles. A quarter of them died from complications. Next to it was a ward packed with tuberculosis patients getting their daily injections for a month or longer.

I saw diseases I never treated in training. I still hear the paroxysms of whooping cough and see the convulsive spasms of tetanus. It broke my heart to see neonates die because their umbilical cord was cut with a dirty garden knife. Severe worm manifestations were so common we frequently operated to remove a large wiggly bolus of roundworms causing a bowel obstruction.

Add to that list marasmus, kwashiorkor, severe scabies, deaths from rabies, anthrax from eating raw liver from cows that died from the disease, leeches on the eyeball, malaria, dengue fever, hydatid cysts, amebic abscesses and a host of other preventable diseases. As we treated a never-ending parade of pathology, it soon became obvious that not long after we sent a patient home, that same patient was back with the same or another preventable disease. Sooner or later, something would take their life.

The problem seemed insurmountable. With only three doctors and six trained nurses, we were overwhelmed. We were so overwhelmed that the nurses were covering the hospital at night in addition to doing all the routine deliveries. We were on a treadmill going faster and faster in a country with the highest population growth in the world. We were going to finally fly off the end of the speeding belt and hit the wall if we didn't do something.

Fast forward just six years. Hospital statistics and disease patterns were dramatically changing due to a grassroots community-based healthcare program funded with secular money and requiring only one missionary nurse's full-time involvement. The program was so innovative and successful that the American ambassador as well as healthcare professionals from 18 difference countries visited us to learn the secrets.

I say that not to blow anyone's horn but to make this point. I don't know the particulars of your present or future situation, but I know you can help people to be much healthier with a minimal investment of staff. Whether you are envisioning beginning a program or already have one started, I'm going to share some principles that can turbo-charge your program. I want you to know how a community health program can be your greatest tool for evangelism and church growth, and you don't need a master's in public health to do it. You will learn how to motivate volunteers to help them be successful throughout the long haul and find out the secret of getting other people to fund your project.

Get Stakeholders' Buy In

There is often tension between those involved in curative and pre-ventative outreaches. I know them well. Some hardcore community health purists maintain that prevention is more cost effective, requires fewer resources, and is a better way to impact the community, all of which are true. But then they assert that curative outreaches should be abandoned. Of course, that is ridiculous. Community health can't cure appendicitis or prevent 100 percent of diseases. Both preventative and curative services are needed, just like two arms are needed to carry a log. They complement and enhance each other. They need each other. Either alone is like a one-armed wallpaper hanger.

Start out by seeking an understanding of an equal partnership. In the early stages, it is common for the overworked curative side to get strapped for staff and then demand the nurse or doctor involved in community health come back to help meet the urgent need "temporarily." Head this off at the pass by agreeing to take that option off the table before the issue even arises. Community health needs a full-time champion fully dedicated to making it happen.

The community health side of the equation needs to recognize that the hospital or health center's good reputation is an enormous asset to what they are trying to accomplish. It saves years of time building credibility and trust in the community. In most instances, it is a great advantage to be seen as an extension of that known ministry. It also makes it much easier to get funding as the program isn't seen as a risky startup without a history.

Don't forget to get support from other stakeholders. The national church is a major exponent. Take the time to discuss your plans and dreams with the national church leaders. Seek their advice and input. Deal with the sticky issue of whether this is going to be a church program limited to their members or a true community-owned program. Make the point that even the community health group you are starting is merely a facilitator and doesn't own the program. The local people do as they are the ones doing most of the work. Remind church officials that the program can be a phenomenal church growth tool, and that they also don't have to own or limit it to get the benefit they desire.

Depending on your location situation, you may need to secure the support of government officials. If nothing else, make a courtesy call to those overseeing your proposed service area. You are going to need their goodwill and cooperation.

I've learned that the key to keeping stakeholders happy is to give the credit away. Use every opportunity to laud your stakeholders as the program succeeds. You will get a huge return on your investment if you use public meetings, letters, and phone calls to make them look good. The more credit you give away, the more it boomerangs back as others say good things about you.

Imitation is the Nicest Form of Flattery
I knew nothing about community health when Susan Carter and I started our community health program. We read books and articles

as we contemplated our startup and then developed a list of all the questions we had and decisions we were going to have to make:

1. Should it be a church, hospital, or community program?
2. Should it be volunteer-based or should we pay our community health workers?
3. Do we need trained supervisors or can we train them ourselves?
4. Do women or men make the best community workers?
5. Do we call them workers or something else? Does the term "workers" communicate the idea of a salaried position?
6. Who should select our community committees? And how should they be chosen? How big should they be?
7. What training will they need?
8. How and where should we train our volunteers?
9. How often do they need supervision?
10. How do we avoid dropout?

And that was just the beginning. If I remember right, we had eight pages of questions ranging from what sort of transport we should buy, to what topics we should teach, to asking other groups where they were getting funding. After much discussion that led to few answers, we made our smartest move. We scheduled two one-week periods away from the hospital and tried to visit as many community health programs as possible. With our questionnaire in hand, we spent time asking specific questions, as well as general inquiries that helped us troll for difficulties we might not have considered ourselves such as:

1. What are your biggest problems?
2. What would you do differently if you started over today?
3. What are the three most important things we need to know to be successful?
4. How are your relationships with your stakeholders? What has gone well and not gone so well? Why?

We even mailed our questions out to those programs we couldn't visit to ensure we had as much information as possible. We then sat down and reviewed the answers, dividing the remaining issues into three categories:

1. It is obvious this solutions works for this issue, and we should do it the same way the vast majority found successful.
2. The answer is not as obvious, but here is what seems to work best. How can we tweak this solution to make it better?
3. All of the programs have this problem, but no one has found the answer. What solution can we come up with?

Let me give you an example. We asked how often each program provided supervision for its volunteer Community Health Helpers (CHHs), and most programs tried to do it once a month. When we asked them to clarify the word "tried," we learned it was actually only every two or three months at best for a litany of reasons mainly involving transportation. "The Land Rover is in the shop. The Bishop needs the vehicle. The Land Rover can't get to that site because the roads are so bad. We don't have the money for the fuel for the vehicle. Someone else in our program needed the Land Rover." Vehicles had a 100 percent import duty and were so expensive that most groups only had one. We learned that those employees hired to supervise and motivate the CHHs spent the vast majority of time sitting in their offices. Visits were sporadic and infrequent; as a result, programs were losing volunteers because of it.

Realizing that volunteers required more supervision than paid staff, we did something no one else had done. We didn't buy a Land Rover; instead, we bought each supervisor a motorcycle designed for herding sheep in the Australian outback. They were built like tanks with protective bars around all vital components with powerful engines, huge knobby tires to move more easily through mud, and platforms behind the driver's seat for transporting goods.

We told our salaried supervisors we expected them to be out in the community four and a half days each week with only a half day in the office to get caught up on paperwork. They were expected to meet with each of their CHHs three times a month. During their first year or two, they were expected to spend two to three hours individually with each CHH each month visiting homes. At the first home, the supervisor would do a home assessment, teach, and share a witness. They would discuss what happened after leaving the home. At the next hut, the CHH would do the visit, allowing the supervisor to critique the performance and point out ways for improvement. This modeling and teaching technique fostered rapid improvement in the first year or so after CHHs received training.

The supervisor would also meet with their CHHs at the monthly community health committee meeting and the monthly immunization clinic the supervisor held in each community. Frequent supervision, role modeling, and deep relationships including praying together fostered extraordinary achievement and low dropout rates as each CHH gave two half-days each week to help their neighbors.

We would not have come up with half of our ideas if we hadn't taken the time to learn from other programs' successes and mistakes. It enabled us to avoid many pitfalls and our new program took off like a racehorse. It is always easier to do it right the first time than to changes horses in the middle of the stream.

It is never too late to learn from others even if you have already started your program. Take the time to visit other groups. If others come to visit you, pick their brains and continue to learn. You are either getting smarter or you are getting dumber.

Get Training of Trainers (TOT) Education
In our medical training, the worst types of educational techniques were applied to us. Lecture is a great way to dump large quantities of information quickly on students, but most of the information goes in one ear and out the other at light speed. Students have to go back and memorize much of their notes or digest a textbook to be able to spit back the information they were given. They cram for the test and then quickly forget much of what they "learned." It is unlikely there will be any changes in behavior even if the information truck dumped on them.

How many lessons have you heard about eating a balanced diet, exercising regularly, or getting adequate sleep? You can quote the data to others who themselves are unlikely to change because of it. That is because God didn't design people that way. We are more likely to change behavior when we are emotionally moved as we learn. This not only better imprints information but also motivates change. Adults learn better through humor, stories, skits, songs, pictures, and other psychosocial teaching methods.

Let me give you an example. If you can convince people to use a clean water source, you will save lives. You could prepare a lecture, show pictures of bacteria, display graphs of cases of diarrhea from drinking river water, and share drawings of fences protecting springs. It is unlikely that much will change after people thank you for bringing your presentation to the village. Here is one way we taught the subject of clean water.

Our local CHHs would take a donkey to the river and get a barrel of water. On the hillside in the village they would use a hoe to dig a shallow ditch down a small hill in the village and then dig a little pool at the end of it. Along the ditch they would place broken tree limbs to imitate trees and bushes and put a sign up saying, "The Nyangores River," the river that most of the people got their water from. The CHHs then invited the village people to watch as water was poured into the ditch.

First, a female CHH would come to the river while carrying a child on her back, her dirty clothes under her arm, and a box of "Omo," the local laundry soap, in her hands. The river would quickly fill with soap suds that washed down to the pool at the end as she washed the laundry.

Then a man would come pulling his cow to water it. The cow would dislodge lots of dirt, sticks, and leaves into the "river." The next man to arrive would look around pretending to find a private spot and then urinate in the "river." Well, at least it looked like that as he used water in a squirt bottle hidden under a blanket draped around him. Finally the last man would come holding his stomach in obvious pain. He would kneel by the river and appear to have diarrhea into the water flowing down the ditch.

By this time, the women in the audience would be throwing their wraps over their heads, shaking with embarrassment and laughter. Another CHH actress would arrive, dipping some water from the pool, taking it to her "husband" sitting on a log by a fire, and giving him a drink. Within minutes after taking a drink, he would be yelling in pain and holding his abdomen while his "neighbors" put him on a stretcher and took him to the hospital with much shouting and consternation.

Then one of the volunteers would ask the jabbering crowed some questions. "What did you see?" He thanked the attendees for their responses until all the elements of the skit were identified. Then he asked the question, "Do these things happen in the river where you get your water?" When the community people said "yes," the next question was, "What was the problem?" That is when things normally started to get interesting. Eventually someone would say, "The water made him sick." Thanking the person for that answer, the CHH then asked "Why did the water make him sick?"

Someone yelled out, "There was too much sugar in his tea!" Other responses also missed the point until someone said, "I think the water was dirty. I've heard that the river water has small animals in it that can make you sick." After discussion, everyone agrees. The next question would be, "How can you get water to drink that does not contain the animals that make you sick?" Someone may state they know someone who gets their water from a spring and they don't seem to get sick. Other attendees may admit they don't have a spring.

Then someone would say that they know people who boil the water to kill the animals in it that make you sick. When people agreed that could help, the question was asked, "How should you boil the water?" and the whole group would be invited to gather around the fire to see a demonstration on boiling water and protecting it from contamination. Of course, other options for clean water would also be discussed.

The training may take a couple of hours, but no one forgets what they learned and many change their habits. They not only had an emotional experience but they frequently say, "You didn't teach us anything. We taught ourselves."

The TOT course teaches you to think differently, teach in a much more effective way, understand community dynamics, and much more. It is now available all over the world. Check the appendix for organizations where you can get this training.

Your Success Depends on the Quality of the Leaders You Choose
Your job will be incredibly harder or much easier depending on the leaders you choose and train. The first personnel you pick are your

Community Health Supervisors. You may have a pool of formally trained nurses or other professionals to choose from. We didn't. We started with a pool of our best "medicine dispensers," local young men we trained to dispense medications on the ward. We looked for people who were bright, were more spiritually mature than their counterparts, and showed a propensity to learn.

We talked about the problems we saw at the hospital and the causes of those problems. Did they see these problems in the villages where they lived? Were they interested in helping save people's lives by teaching them better health practices? We warned that they would have to work very hard, but we would teach them how to do their job well.

We didn't promise them more money. We let them know we were happy with their work in the hospital; they could continue in their current position and would probably be promoted over time. We didn't want our new supervisors to choose to join us for the wrong reasons. We weren't offering them a different job. Instead, we were offering the opportunity to join our community health family and change their world. We wanted them to sense that God was calling them to this endeavor, so we prayed with them and asked they seek God's will in their decision.

Our first three supervisors were very committed to the idea, but had no experience or knowledge to do the job we needed them to do. It was up to us to turn them into extraordinary leaders and teach them the same lessons we were learning on the job. That meant spending time together letting them watch what did, how we taught, how we developed trust, and how we worked to reveal our servant hearts. We demonstrated leadership and then began to edge them into increasing leadership responsibilities.

We held them accountable with job descriptions and clear standards of performance. How were they going to know they were doing each item of the job description well? As their supervisors, what measurements showed us that they were meeting all of their responsibilities? We set up one-on-one evaluation times on a regular basis and clearly let them know what they were doing well and where they needed to improve.

We invested a great deal of time supplying knowledge as well as modeling every aspect of what we wanted them to do. As they made progress, we morphed our methods. We sat down with all of the supervisors every morning before they headed into the community and asked each to answer some simple but broad questions:

- What went well yesterday? What progress are you seeing in those you supervise?
- What problems did you have? What didn't go well?
- How can you solve these problems?

We let each individual answer and then threw the most perplexing problems out to the other supervisors for input. We taught them to work as a team, help each other out, and share what they learned with others. As much as possible, we didn't prescribe solutions. We wanted to teach our young leaders how to solve problems by planning concrete steps to deal with them and then finding out how their plans worked. We even listed major problems on plastic sheets hanging on the wall to remind us to follow-up in future sessions.

I can teach someone all the reasons and benefits of exercising, demonstrate how to use exercise machines, and share knowledge on how to do reps; however, until they actually get on the machines and workout, they won't strengthen a muscle. The same is true in leadership training. You have to give those you are mentoring ever-increasing leadership responsibilities as they develop. You have to be present on the sidelines coaching and teaching them how to solve problems, motivate people, take risks, deal with discouragement, and become a coach themselves. It is all about replication as you train leaders to train more leaders for your community health committees and volunteers.

As I look back now years later, I'm so glad I invested in these young men and the other workers who later joined them. Not only were they one of the keys to our success, but they each are now in major leadership positions in other spheres of life. Some are chiefs or assistant chiefs, others have positions in the national church, and some have been successful in politics. More importantly, they changed their communities through their faithful service and leadership. That is a wonderful return on our investment.

Leadership training is a journey, not an event. It is a demonstration, not just an education. It is learning to influence others, not merely having position over them. It is building trust, respect, and admiration.

If You Haven't Measured It, You Haven't Done It
What have you really accomplished through your efforts? That is a huge question you, and especially present and prospective funders, want to know. Are your investments in planning and execution bringing dividends? How big of a dividend? What is working and what is not? What do you need to change to make what is not working actually work? So what do you measure? You need to decide that first. What are the key indicators to show that you are lowering morbidity and mortality? What things need to happen to demonstrate that you are successful in making your target populations healthier?

If people build and use pit latrines, studies show there is a decrease in parasite infestations, diarrheal disease, and other problems, so you may want to measure that. If a family has a clean water source they consistently use, they will be healthier and have fewer visits to the clinic or hospital. As a result, you will decrease the cases of dehydration from gastroenteritis, so you may want to measure that. Those are just examples, but whether you are starting a program or enhancing one, you need to determine your key indicators to show you are accomplishing your goals.

Though we were anxious to hit the ground running with our program, we made sure we took the time to complete a crucial task first. We conducted a survey of 600 homes to determine our baseline. We partnered with a U.S. university to ensure the validity of our survey instruments and subsequently do an objective analysis of our data. To avoid surveyor bias, we hired local teachers during their school break to go house to house to collect the information. When we finished, we had great objective data that wasn't available from other sources on subjects like immunization rates, latrines, and a host of other health behaviors we planned to target.

We trained the teachers to administer the survey correctly. How should they ask the questions to ensure each family understood? We asked them to visually confirm the information they were given if at all possible. If they were told the family had a latrine, they needed to verify if it was truly there and if a path was worn from the hut to the toilet. They should examine each child's "Road to Health" immunization card to verify their immunizations, see if the family had a raised fireplace, check if they were boiling their water, and much more. We wanted good data to show where we were so we would clearly see our successes and failures in bringing lasting change to the local community.

We then followed up by completing surveys of 2,000 homes every three years after the program was underway, but we did it with a new twist. We divided those homes into three groups. The first group included homes where our CHHs were teaching and helping their neighbors. The second group included homes with no CHHs, but the homes were located adjacent to where we were working. We were looking for spillover from families who were impacted and then influenced their neighbors who didn't have CHHs. The last group of homes we surveyed was some distance away so it had no program influence. Was our baseline changing over time from other influences?

All of this took time and money, but we built the cost into our funding proposal. The results were more than worth it. We had concrete data to guide our efforts and our funders saw the return on their investment. In fact, the data was so dramatic to USAID that the American ambassador visited the program. Some of the programs we visited before we started our program visited us to learn our methods.

Over time, surveys show change, but a snapshot every three years is not enough. You also need to measure effort and change every month to measure your progress, identify problems, and motivate your staff and volunteers.

It is no different than when you were in school. When the teacher told you that certain information was going to be on the exam you studied and learned it. When a paper was going to be 30 percent of your grade, you focused on doing it well. The same is true with your staff and volunteers, so ask them to report regularly.

What indicates effort? These questions help answer that question, but you may think of others. Are they visiting new homes? Are they revisiting families to teach new concepts? Are they sharing the gospel? Are they working to make their homes good examples?

You also want to measure change because effort is not enough. A CHH may be working hard but is ineffective. That is a red flag to the supervisor to spend time finding out why. Is it their communication technique? Are they teaching the lessons wrong? Are they rushing their engagements? Are they not accepted in their community for some reason?

You will likely have more interventions than you can reasonably ask your volunteers to report on. What are the most important ones for improving health? What are your funders most interested in?

Our program had twenty-five teaching focuses, but the primary purpose of our funding was community distribution of family planning supplies because Kenya had the highest population growth rate in the world at that time. We made sure we did enough measurements in this area to fulfill our obligation to our donor. We then looked at the behaviors causing the most morbidity and mortality and measured those indicators as well. For example, having a clean water source obviously fell into that category. On the other hand, though we taught about having a "hanging wire" (clothes line) versus drying clothes on the ground where they could pick up scabies mites, we didn't measure that since it was of lesser importance.

For reports to be useful, people need to be able to compare their efforts and results with others. If you got an 80 percent on an exam in school, you were either disappointed or elated based on whether that was the lowest or the highest grade in your class! Measurements need context to have significance, so work out some way to report back to your volunteers and supervisors. We did that with a monthly newspaper that contained the eight or ten of the most important indicators for each of our health volunteers. We also printed the total for each committee so they could compare themselves to others. This also gave us a way to monitor the effectiveness of each supervisor as they compared their health helper and committee results with their colleagues.

As you have success in one area that you are measuring and realize an area you are not measuring is not seeing the change you seek, you can change what you report. You will quickly see new effort and change as your volunteers realign their priorities.

Monthly measurements are the speedometer of your program and periodic surveys are the odometer. Don't attempt to drive your program without them.

There is one other easy way to demonstrate your success. Use the annual statistics from your hospital and/or clinics for the diseases you are trying to ameliorate. If you are focusing on clean water, look at your admission statistics for gastroenteritis and dehydration. If you have a low immunization rate and are trying to turbocharge your vaccination program in children, what is happening with admissions for the diseases you are trying to prevent? Take those yearly numbers and graph them over time.

You may even want to do some chart audits for a specific disease. Are your measles cases coming from areas where you have been working or areas you haven't reached yet? Statistics powerfully supplement your surveys and monthly statistics.

Yes, all of this takes time, but it gives you important information to guide your efforts, inform your donors, motivate your team and celebrate your successes.

To Treat or Not to Treat
Another early decision was whether we would train our community volunteers, many with minimal education, to treat common diseases. Here is the decision tree that we climbed down to get to the root of our answer. These questions will assist you in making your decision based on your local conditions.

- Were there significant medical needs in the community? We identified the ten most common easily treatable illnesses, looked at their incident rates in the community, and identified how many patients were admitted to the hospital with complications. We found a significant unmet disease burden.
- Were diagnostic and treatment modalities available on a timely basis? There were few clinics or other places the local

people could get treatment. The few government facilities were poorly staffed, equipped, and supplied. People had to walk long distances to get treatment. "Bush doctors" preyed on their plight by scavenging used vials and empty medicine bottles, stealing medicines, claiming knowledge they did not have, and setting up "practices" in the community. Vials were filled with river water and contaminated syringes and needles were used to give injections again and again. Aspirin was sold as an antibiotic. Dangerous medicines were given with no knowledge of their effects or proper dosage.

- Could we properly train our CHHs? We thought we could if we limited their repertoire to only ten diseases, most of them not requiring dangerous drugs. We realized it was going to take repetitive teaching and then ongoing supervision with frequent monitoring in the field. We decided before we even began that we needed to be ready to abandon this component of the program if it was not working well.
- Could we minimize risks? We identified a number of risks:
  - Our CHHs could give medications when they were not needed or for the wrong condition. Were they diagnosing correctly? We ascertained that one-on-one mentoring was needed during training and the early days in the field so our supervisors could help them apply the newly gained knowledge and observe the results.
  - They could give the wrong dose of medicine. Thirty years ago, malaria could still be treated with chloroquine in our service area, but adult doses given to young children could kill them. To avoid incorrect dosing, we adopted a unit dose packaging system for all our medications. Each envelope was clearly marked with the name of its contents, the expiration date of the medicine, for what age it was appropriate, and how it was to be taken (using symbols for those who could not read).
  - As we had a large problem with corruption, theft, and fraud in our service area, recruiting the right people and good close supervision were obviously the first safeguards, but we wanted to lower temptation with good systems. All pill envelopes were sealed and then enclosed in ziplock bags in groups of ten for easy inventory. Medicines were kept in a large locked wooden "medicine box"

by the local committee. Before new medicines would be issued, the CHHs had to have their medicine bags inventoried to show medicines present or the money they received for them. They turned in the money to get another batch of medications.
- Added Benefits – We did not pay our volunteers, but we realized they would incur expenses as they served. Mothers with children with gastroenteritis would bring them to their homes and they would have to use their own sugar and salt to make oral rehydration solution. Others might desperately need medicine but couldn't afford it. CHHs might be too far from home to return for a meal and have to provide food at a local "duka" (store). For these reasons, we built a small "profit" into their medicines sales. It was not large enough to give a stimulus to sell medicines when they were not needed but high enough to cover some of their expenses.

Overall, our medicine system worked well. It gave our CHHs higher respect in the community as they treated malaria, peptic ulcer disease, small wounds, burns, cough, worms, and other diseases, as well as provided vitamins. A medication distribution system might not make sense in your area so use this decision tree to find out.

Fund Your Program

You can do community health with comparatively little funding compared to curative outreaches, but funding can turbocharge your program when used properly. You can do more and expand quicker. Community health outreach gives a high return on a small investment, but I've never seen a program totally self-supporting. There are costs for supervisors' salaries and benefits, transportation, computers, stationary supplies, training, and more. How do you fund it?

A number of streams are available for funding that should come together to make it happen. Missionary salaries and expenses may come from their ministry accounts, which is a gift in kind to the program though few missionaries are actually involved in the program. In our case, we had only one or two missionaries involved full-time in the early days.

You can generate some income from program activities. Our medication program also included income opportunities for each committee to do local projects and for the central office to help fund activities. This amount wasn't huge, but it was significant in showing outside funders we were doing our part to fund our work. Our hospital provided some services gratis, another gift in kind.

What we did not generate from medication sales, we raised from mission funds to help cover the cost of our evangelism and discipleship efforts including purchasing Bibles, tracts, and other materials and to cover the cost of spiritual training for CHHs. We wanted to show our secular funders that we weren't using their funds for "proselytizing."

The vast majority of our funds came from project grants we received from government and parastatal organizations. My philosophy is not to use the Lord's money for things the secular world will pay for as long as there are no strings attached to impede our ministry goals. We initially got USAID funds for two three-year cycles of funding. When the U.S. threatened to withhold aid funds to Kenya over political issues, we approached EZE (now EED), a large German parastatal that helped us on other projects. They helped hold us accountable to accomplish what we set out to do, an added bonus to receiving the funding!

You Don't Want to Own It
It is better to have a friend who owns a truck than it is to own it yourself! If you own it, you have all the problems associated with ownership, yet most people only occasionally need a truck for hauling. It is much easier to put some gas in the truck and return it.

The same is true in community health work. You want to indigenize your program. It often takes time to fully nationalize your community-based outreaches, but the process should start from day one. Not only do you need a great deal of input to understand community problems, but you must also give the local health committees the latitude to make decisions and even mistakes as they work. Your central efforts need to be seen as facilitation of the community's efforts so the local people, government officials, and others see "your" program as their program. How do you make that happen?

First, send the right messages and back them up. We told our local committees that the program belonged to them and they made the decisions. Preceding that, we had many discussions about concerns with that strategy. Should we make it a church-based program? We didn't because we thought it would limit our target audience to our own church denomination members. Should we limit it to committee members, health helpers or Christians? That was a harder question. If we did, we would still be holding "veto" power over local decisions. After lots of prayer and discussion, we didn't. Instead, we worked hard to help local councils come to that decision. We had a few trainees come through who really didn't know Christ as their savior, but they came to Christ during training with prayer and testimony.

It is not easy to give up control but it pays off in many different ways. If you use volunteers, sooner or later some of them will ask to be paid, especially if you are associated with a hospital or have outside funding from a grant-making organization. The problem is not hard to handle if you have truly made your local committees in charge. You just tell the volunteer that they need to talk to the local committee since they are in charge. Politics exist in every country and community. As someone from another country, you don't completely understand the local politics and you definitely don't want to get into the middle of it. It is much better if the local committees deal with those issues.

True indigenization is like raising kids. To teach them responsibility, you set them increasingly free with more and more responsibility. The same is true in emancipating your local committees from central support. As they learn to motivate, train, equip, supervise, and hold people accountable, you can step further and further back from the process, giving less and less of your resources from your central office. Do this slowly but methodically based on performance, not time. Is this local committee solving problems, showing initiative, and managing its people well? As they prove themselves, you step back and become the encourager, providing advice only as it is requested. At the same time, you praise them for their accomplishments and give them credit with others for their successes.

Focus on the Eternal
Community health is one of the best methods for evangelism, discipleship, and fueling church growth. It combines the effective synergy

of words and works with an "every person" campaign as your health helpers draw maps of their communities and visit every home.

Here are the "Ps" of an effective program:

- Passion – If you are directing the program, the passion has to first be manifested in you. Remember, no matter how much you improve health behaviors, sooner or later every person is going to die. The only way you can provide eternal life is to introduce people to Christ. So you need to practice what you preach in your words and deeds. Be more excited about this part of training than anything else you do. Your passion will be contagious. Get out in front and demonstrate how to do it while others watch. You can be involved in evangelism skits or take individual health helpers with you on home visits to demonstrate how you share your faith.

  Let your supervisors know this is the most important thing they need to facilitate. Disciple and mentor them so they can disciple and mentor those they supervise. Hold them accountable by direct observation and through their reports. Provide feedback and continuing education to constantly stimulate them to do better.

  Collect data on your evangelism outreach. Measure both your efforts and your results. How many people did each health helper share the gospel with last month? How many people came to Christ? How many of those people are now incorporated in a local church? Collect testimonies of those who came to Christ and share it with all your staff and volunteers.

  The Holy Spirit is the only one who can convict and bring someone to repentance. Pray and encourage everyone to bathe the community health teams' efforts in prayer. You have not because you ask not, so ask in faith believing and then do the work. Keep your church leaders up to date on your efforts and results. Let them know that you are there to complement and supplement their efforts. Your goal is to help them be more successful. As God works, give the credit away to others, realizing that only through His grace is anything accomplished.

- Plan – Things rarely happen by accident. You need to create a plan and continually sharpen it to make it better. Develop culturally appropriate methods for sharing the gospel in a wide range of situations. What skits or stories will share your message effectively? How can you use a picture or have your health helpers draw a diagram to explain salvation? What cultural practices, beliefs, or stories can be used to find bridges to share biblical truths?

  Test each method you develop to see what works best. Turn your supervisors and helpers loose to be creative. Before long, you will have as effective or even more effective methods for evangelism as you have for your health interventions. Don't forget to talk to other groups to learn from them and share your methods.

- Purpose – You wouldn't deliver a baby in the hospital and leave it in the delivery room forever. If you did, sooner or later it would perish for lack of food, warmth, and love. No, you place the swaddled child into her mother's arms, ensure that she nurses, and then give the new mom instructions.

  In the same way, it is important for your community health team to know their ultimate purpose is to build the church. It is the church that can help new Christians mature in their faith. As people come to Christ, they may be involved in some of the early discipleship efforts, but they need to have close relationships with the local church and get new converts participating as soon as possible. That is where they will grow, develop, and find the support structures they need to become all God designed them to be.

You may run into the problem we did. We found the local church poorly trained and equipped to disciple thousands of new converts each year. We recruited a long time missionary and doctor's wife who volunteered to train pastors in the areas where we were working. She held mini-pastors' conferences that taught a new believer training curriculum we developed. From this point of contact, we developed long-term relationships with individual pastors and checked back with them regularly to see how they were doing and encourage them in their efforts. We funded and provided Bibles and discipleship materials as needed.

We found our community health program to be a massive generator for church growth. We peaked at close to 10,000 new converts a year.

Clone It

Okay, I'm not for human cloning, but cloning program principles makes sense. Our community health program gave us a laboratory for testing and developing management methods, fundraising processes, logistical systems, training approaches, and motivational techniques. What a waste to only utilize what we learned within that one program.

We soon realized two things. Our health outreach mainly transformed women and children. We were not reaching men very often. Secondly, money had a lot to do with health. We could teach proper nutrition, but the family couldn't afford to buy what they needed if they didn't have the financial resources. They also couldn't afford school fees, clothes, clinic fees, etc. At the same time, men were interested in making money.

We already had the systems and methods developed from our health efforts, so we simply cloned our program into a development outreach with different interventions. We went looking and found the best micro-enterprise methods that we felt could be even better. Instead of working to create interest in new enterprises, we focused on how we could make the local people very successful in what they already knew. We focused in four areas.

First, we taught and modeled "zero-grazing" to increase milk and calf production. We motivated men to sell all but the best three or four cows, contain them in a feeding shed, and grow high protein fodder on their limited land. They brought the cows water from the river on a donkey so they wouldn't "walk off" their milk production or get diseases from other cows in the community. They cut the fodder, brought it to the cows, and saw their milk production soar. We got the government to bring in artificial insemination services to help breed better cows. We worked to set up local collection systems for our milk producers.

In our African culture, women did the gardening. We worked with a U.S.-based company to build greenhouses and grow hybrid plants that markedly increased production. We then helped finance smaller satellite greenhouses in local communities run by our health committees. This ensured vegetables for each family and they had enough to sell and generate income. Along with this, we provided cheap "bucket-based" drip irrigation systems for drier areas.

Chickens were a great source of protein through their eggs and ultimately meat. Most bush hens free ranged and had poor egg production if they could be found in the weeds. We developed a "no touch" of the ground chicken coop for twenty hens to prevent disease transmission, set up brooder houses for hybrid high production layer hens, and developed chicken feed distribution systems. In fifteen minutes, a woman could feed and water her hens and collect around fifteen eggs a day which were readily marketable. Lastly, we developed a rain water containment system made out of readily available local materials that supplied a source of safe water for families.

We trained men to teach development and used the same techniques we perfected in our health work. We also constructed demonstration projects where the lessons being taught could be demonstrated.

And we didn't stop there. As our reputation grew, we cloned our techniques back into our hospital, clinics, the new nursing school, and even the church administration. For example, we learned from using skits that we could teach as well as assess what our health and development helpers really knew. So we incorporated role playing into our nursing student interviewing process. We would ask an applicant to pretend one of the interviewers was a family member of a patient who had just died on the ward and ask them relate that fact in a compassionate manner. We might ask them to act out sharing the gospel with a patient, deal with a colleague who wasn't doing their job well, or participate in a half dozen other scenarios which gave us insight into their ability to think, communication skills, maturity, or knowledge base.

So how do I sum it up? Community health outreaches are "high leverage." You get a lot of "bang" for your buck! Limited resources can bring enormous results. Preventing disease is so much better than treating, and community health programs bring long-lasting changes in behavior. Most importantly, they are one of the best ways to spread the gospel.

If you don't have a program, start one. If you have an outreach, turbocharge it by applying some of these techniques. People will be glad you did!

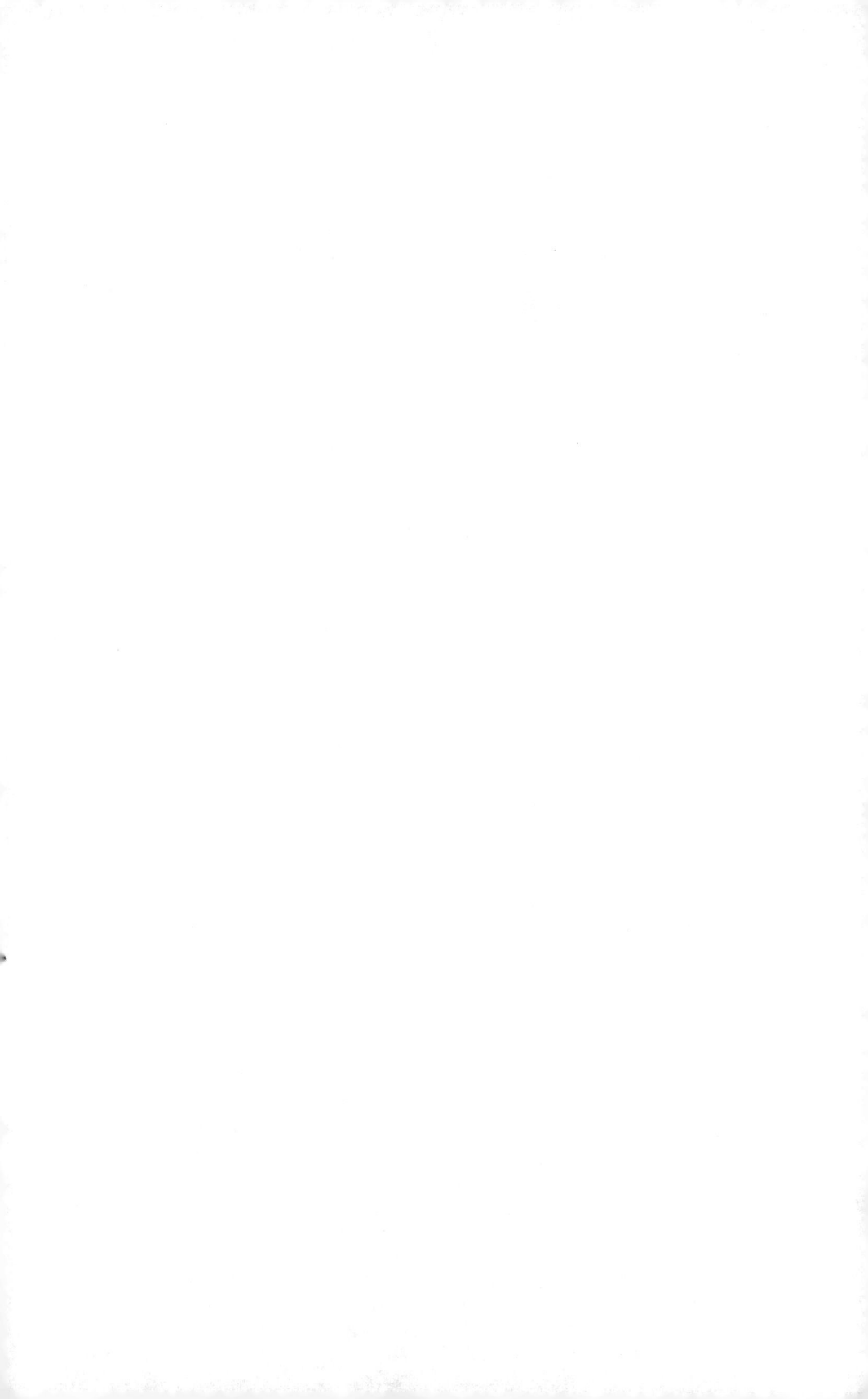

CHAPTER 31
TRAIN UP

Aristotle once said, "Excellence is an art won by training." You will never change the overall health of your patients without proper training. No matter how hard you labor, you will just be filling a bucket with water that has a hole in the bottom.

Community health evangelism is the ideal way to prevent disease as you teach people better health practices while changing their minds and hearts. Nevertheless, that still leaves the curative side of the equation including the employees working in your hospital, clinic, or other institution. No matter how reliable your prevention training, people are still going to get appendicitis, cancer, and a host of other diseases needing treatment. And that means you are going to need trained staff to help cure their ailments.

In pioneer curative medical missions, training is traditionally done on the job with short courses and lots of hands-on mentoring. When I arrived at Tenwek, we had "ward attendants" who were hired, attended some basic classes, and then assigned duties such as moving patients, sweeping floors, changing beds, and various other duties. The best were promoted to become "medicine dispensers" and were trained to dispense medicines and give injections on the ward. In those early days, we only had six or seven nurses with formal training who focused on supervision, diagnosis, treatment, and midwifery. It was the best that could be done with our available resources, but it was far from the excellence we wanted. I still remember trying to teach an illiterate mother how to suction her three-year-old son's tracheostomy during the night when only one trained nurse was available for the entire hospital. On the second night, exhausted, she fell asleep and the child obstructed and died.

Essentially, we had the chicken and the egg problem. We needed nurses, but we were stymied because we didn't have enough nurses to open a training school. We also didn't have enough doctors, lab techs, chaplains, and other professional staff. We needed a nursing school in the worst way, but how could we afford to spend the time to start it when we were already in such desperate straits? We also needed laboratory, chaplaincy, community health, and other training programs. I could perform quick C-sections or see seventy-five to one hundred patients a day, but that wasn't going to solve our basic problems. We needed trained and fully committed healthcare professionals.

That is why I was involved in starting three training schools that produced excellent graduates who transformed our work and the work of others. Out of dozens of schools in the country, Tenwek's nursing school had three of the top ten students on the national exam a few years ago. Training continues to expand; today, there is also family practice training and a surgical residency program.

Looking back, training was the most strategic thing we did to improve the health of our constituency. Like having children, reproduction and multiplication influence lives long after the "parent" moves out of the scene. And as I watch today's mission healthcare landscape around the world, it is evident that training has the longest and largest impact. Larger mission facilities are increasingly moving into residency training. So what are the key principles to starting and then running a good training program?

Strategize
Strategically decide what training programs you need. Also prioritize them. You probably can't do all the programs at once so start with the program most needed.

Plan
To start planning a program, begin by completing a strengths and weaknesses analysis. What supplies or resources do you already have to facilitate this training program? Review your staff, patient load, facilities, applicant pools, funding streams, teachers, networks, government contacts for accreditation, etc. Many of these issues will likely fall into your weakness category. At Tenwek, we had a great need

for nurses and plenty of patients, but not much else. We were concerned it might even be difficult to find qualified applicants because the schools were so poor in our area. Even if we did find applicants, we worried how we could keep the graduates when they were so concerned about their own children's educational opportunities. We added that latter issue to our list of weaknesses.

Once you've completed the analysis, divide your list of weaknesses into three categories:

- Items that have to be solved in order to start a program.
- Items that need to be solved, but can happen over time.
- Items that would be helpful to have solved, but aren't necessary to start a program.

Go for It

It is easy to look at this problem list of weaknesses, conclude it's too difficult, and decide to simply give up on making the needed changes. As with all problems, the mountain can seem too high. Remember, you don't have to jump over the mountain all at once, but can just climb it one step at a time. Consider the rewards that will come with this accomplishment, have a time of prayer and fasting, seek God's guidance, and obey His leading. He has all the resources in the world. If He says "go," then go for it.

Harness the Team

Committees waste a considerable amount of time, but a core group of people needs to be brought together as a task force to get the work accomplished. Organize the task force by casting the vision and getting commitments from each person. This task force may only be two to five people. A bloated task force does not run well, so you want the fewest number of people who can accomplish the goal. More than likely, many other people will just need to be kept informed instead of actually being on the task force.

Overcome Obstacles

Prioritize all of the items on your list of weaknesses that have to be solved in order to start a program. What are the choke points and the release points? For example, your task force has so many individual responsibilities that it would be helpful to hire a key leader of the training school in the early stages to handle much of the work needing to be done. Filling that position would turn a potential choke point into a release point. Let's dig into some of the common issues in starting a training institution.

- *School leader*. Training schools rarely rise above the quality of the key leader. That person sets the tone for excellence, hard work, good management, while serving as a role model for the students and faculty. Hiring this person should be high on your priority list. Perhaps you have a person who already understands the culture, knows your work, has the credentials, and can be relieved from their present responsibilities to focus on this new task. That is the ideal situation, but is often not the case. Instead, you have to search for someone to fill the position. A common mistake is to simply "make do" with what you have available. If it works at all, you will probably end up with more problems and poorer products. Without the right leader, you will waste precious time and money that could be better used elsewhere. Pray, be patient, and search for the right leader. It is the first key to success. Remember these principles:
  - Develop your dream qualifications. What is the profile of an individual who could really make this training school successful?
  - Make a short list of qualified individuals. Spread the word about what type of leader you are looking for as far and wide as you can. Ask people to suggest applicants they think may qualify for the position.
  - You have not because you ask not. The tendency is to leave recruiting to your mission agency or just wait on the Lord. You need to do your part. During our nursing school project at Tenwek, I spread the word and heard about a missionary nurse in Papua, New Guinea, who had degrees in both nursing and midwifery, as well as a great interest in education. She was also considering a venue change from her current workplace. After receiving letters and having a personal conversation with my boss and me, she prayed, considered the opportunity, and ultimately accepted the position. Since then, she has earned multiple other degrees including a doctorate in nursing. The school she leads at Tenwek is considered one of the

best in the country, and she is the primary reason for the school's success over the last few decades. You are a part of God's plan for calling others to assist you.

- *School Size*. Ask yourself what size school you need now, in five years and in ten years. How do other schools retain graduates and what is the success rate? Build a cushion into the program in case you underestimate. This will give you guidance on the size of student housing, classrooms, and faculty. If you are creating great graduates, it will be a blessing to many even if they don't work in your healthcare system long term. On the other hand, each student educated is an investment and your institution needs a return on that. In the African context, each student was "bonded" to the organization for a period of time after graduation. This ensured they all stayed initially and also gave us an opportunity to select those performing best after graduation for longer contracts.

- *Facilities*. You often need dormitories, classrooms, and offices to start a training school. Obviously, you need additional funds to build these necessary facilities. This money problem is often the easiest one to solve. Supporters easily grasp the vision of training nationals, but you also need to think outside the box and approach foundations, para-government organizations, and major donors. Use the online Foundation Directory to search for foundations interested in education in your part of the world. Approach fundraising like a capital campaign and offer naming opportunities for buildings, classrooms, the library, and even the entire school. Major donors often want to honor a loved one and will contribute at a higher level if given the opportunity to memorialize someone.

- *Government accreditation*. I have seen two common mistakes in this arena:
    - Ignoring It. Too many facilities don't go through the work and frustration of getting accredited. This leaves your graduates hamstrung and can end up causing you problems with the authorities. They may ignore it because they think it is too hard or impossible to acquire. Occasionally, it is impossible. Most often, accreditation is pos-

sible to obtain through work and persistence. It is worth the effort if you want to be seen as excellent in the eyes of the medical community and keep up with ever-changing requirements. You also owe it to your trainees. Remember, you can have a great testimony to others involved in the same sort of training if God blesses your new outreach. Accreditation puts you in touch with others doing the same projects and is a great witness.
- Aiming too high. You may have to start at the bottom and work your way up. At Tenwek, we started with an enrolled community nurse school and then worked our way up to a registered level. We would have never qualified for the latter when we first started. Start humbly asking for assistance and approval. Be willing to take advice and act upon it. Work like it all depends on you and trust knowing it all depends on God.

- *Operational costs*. Hiring personnel and building space is only part of the issue. You have to fund the operation of the school. Some of that can be done through student fees, but not even schools in the U.S. can survive on tuition income alone. You will need to raise funds for scholarships, ongoing overhead costs, national teacher salaries, library acquisitions, transportation, and much more. The groups that are successful at this type of fundraising personalize their efforts by clearly breaking down what a donation is for and what it will accomplish. Focus much more of your time on monthly or quarterly gifts through regular electronic deductions than on one-time gifts. Once they setup a regular donation, people will often continue to donate for many years to come.

You may want to consider a formal relationship with a similar Christian school in the U.S. to help provide advice, short-term faculty, and even resources. These sister school relationships also help provide valuable recruiting networks if you offer opportunities for their students to visit and participate at your institution. They also help with publicity since their constituency is regularly informed of the sister school's activities.

Another way to deal with these funding needs is to get your

most ardent supporters involved in establishing a council, board, or foundation in your country of origin that works to promote the school and raise funds. PAACS did that for the mission hospitals it works with, and the organization provides scholarship money, offers oversight, works on accreditation, recruits visiting staff, obtains long-term missionaries, and holds joint conferences. As a result, it performs a large portion of the work individual institutions would normally have to bear which in turn provides a great economy of scale.

Remember to think big enough. The tendency is to underestimate costs, facilities, funding, staffing, and the list goes on. Attempt great things if you know God laid this project on your heart. People are attracted to a bigger vision much more than a smaller one. You want something that is worth investing time, energy, and funds.

- *Institutional changes.* You may have to do significant revamping in your institution to meet accreditation requirements. At Tenwek, we ran our hospital based on our American background. When we started our nursing school, we had to convert the entire institution over to Kenyan standards which were grounded in English traditions. For the first time, nurses had to wear caps and doctors were expected to wear ties. We weren't allowed to dispense medicines from a small cup, but had to design a rolling cart of medications so each person could get their medicines dispensed from a marked original container. We had to create portable privacy screens to be used on the wards and the list went on. Some schools require more institutional changes than others, but modifications in facilities and protocols were required even when we started our laboratory technician and chaplaincy training schools.

- *Equipment and Books.* This is of lesser importance than many of the other factors. With the right leadership and the right product, the necessary tools and equipment will naturally flow to it. But to get started, you will need the basics appropriate to your needs, culture, and space limitations. The good news is that supporters get excited about training nationals, as do corporations and foundations that realize this is the key to sustainability and quality. Just don't allow people to donate "junk for Jesus" on you. Carefully screening gifts is important. For books, visit *www.intlbookproject.org* to learn about the International Book Project. They have good, used, and next to the last edition textbooks and will ship overseas. We used these resources to start a hospital staff recreation-reading library and to help national students in our area schools.

Running the School

Let me touch on just a few things regarding a topic that could fill pages.

- *Student policies.* Take the time to write effective student policy manuals. Start this process by obtaining manuals from other schools in your country. Ask faculty at other schools what they would do differently if they started over again and what problems occurred that they didn't have a policy for. Avoid making the same mistakes by preparing useful and helpful policies for all likely contingencies. What if students can't pay their fees? What is the penalty for cheating? What spiritual instruction are you going to incorporate and how will it be evaluated?

    Character is even more important than knowledge. Just ask employers. It is not so much what is poured into students but what is planted. You need to train people who will be leaders in their profession, giving them even more influence with others. You want to teach, model, and facilitate leadership development. By doing so, your graduates will influence many more people.

    An education system is poor if it only teaches students to make a living without teaching them how to make a life. You want each graduate to have a solid Christian character based on biblical truths. If that is important enough to be made a goal, it is important enough to prioritize in both the teaching and experiences. If you are training in a mission facility, you really want graduates to be medical or dental missionaries themselves wherever they work or whatever they do. You have the unique opportunity to teach competency, as well as disciple them into a deeper relationship with God.

- *Interviews*. We had several discussions about how to acquire the kind of students we wanted. We decided to review more than grades, test scores, and recommendations by conducting interviews. Our interview process gave us the most unusual insights. We asked interviewees to share their testimonies to examine their spiritual maturity and commitment. We also examined the issue of wisdom in decision making by incorporating role playing exercises into the interview process.

  We would give applicants a scenario and ask them to respond and act it out. We would then add various layers of complexity to the situation based on how the applicant performed. We would look for empathy, compassion, spiritual ministry, judgment, wisdom, etc. To alleviate interviewer bias and control other factors, each candidate was interviewed by two different interviewer teams. We felt this unusual interview technique gave us important insights.

- *Retention*. How do you keep your graduates? You have poured funds and time into them. Their excellent training will have other institutions vying to hire them. Some of them may have more resources or other factors to tear them away. One way to handle this is to "bond" students as they arrive for training. With this policy, students agree to work for two years at the hospital on graduation or face a substantial financial penalty. Such a policy has a provision where you can release graduates from bonds if you feel they would not make good employees or if you have problems during their service period. This protocol also gives you a chance to decide whether you want an individual graduate at your institution long-term.

There is no question establishing a training school is a long process requiring a great amount of work. As you go through this process, always remember to pray. Pray for the assurance that God has directed you to start this training school, for wisdom in designing and organizing it, and for the right leader to make it work. Pray for the finances and the new relationships needed to make it successful. Commit the whole project to the Lord and rest in Him.

You will have the longest impact in your country of service through training. As you teach, mentor, and model, you will create a legacy and a benefit to last many years after you depart the scene.

PART 9
FAMILY FOCUS

CHAPTER 32
FAMILY MATTERS

A total of two-thirds of medical students, residents, and young doctors called to missions have anywhere from "concern" to "great fear" of raising their children overseas, according to a survey completed by CMDA's Center for Medical Missions.

I understand. When Jody and I were preparing for a missionary career, our children's education was the biggest issue. At that time, children at our hospital were sent to a boarding school five hours away beginning in the second grade. Even though we wouldn't face that issue in our first term, it was something we discussed and began to make contingency plans for. Homeschooling was in its infancy back then, but we were early accepters! We homeschooled, helped start a one-room school house, and told our children they could go to boarding school when they were ready. They made that plea and went in fifth and sixth grade.

Of course, education is just one of the issues in raising your family and being the husband or wife God wants you to be overseas. I realize every situation is different. You may be in a mega-city where the issues are dissimilar from those in the bush hospital where I served. All the same, I think many of the issues faced are common to all busy missionary healthcare personnel. Here are some principles that may be helpful as you endeavor to make your career and your life "family friendly."

<u>Give It Time</u>
Time is your most rationed commodity, but there is no generic alternative for it. Your spouse and your children need and value it above everything else. In many ways this is much easier for missionary doc-

tors who live where they work than for physicians in Western countries. Unless there was an emergency, I ate breakfast, lunch, and dinner with my children every day.

Repeated studies show the powerful impact of families having meals together. In the U.S., the risk of early sexual behavior or drug use drops significantly for children as they become teens if families have just five meals together a week. If you can't be home for every meal, prioritize family meal times when you can. The other great advantage you have is children can be more involved in what you are doing in many rural situations. My children used to visit the hospital to ask when I was going to be home for supper. When they got older, they were able to observe procedures. It is important to let your children and spouse see the medical side of your life.

As the children got older, I tried to look for ways to get them involved by taking them on clinic trips, out to the game park when I was taking visitors on a tour, or to speaking engagements. The mission field gives you much more latitude in becoming creative in making time for family. We have a distinct advantage over our Western counterparts in many situations. They may think we live in a "dangerous" jungle, but the jungle they live in is much more dangerous. It is a master at separating the family herd. Everyone heads off in different directions. Moral carnivores are adept in taking down stragglers. Of all the blessings of our missionary life, I thank God most that I got to raise my children on the mission field in their early days.

Specialize
Find ways to make each member of your family feel special. Everyone needs family time, but they also need individual time with you. Your spouse tops the list. That can be a challenge when you can't go on a date to see a movie or out to eat because of a remote location. If you haven't read it, get a copy of *The Five Love Languages*, a book to help you understand the five ways individuals like to feel loved. Figure out your spouse's and your children's love languages and work to make them feel special in their individual language.

Jody likes deep conversations and doing things together. When the hospital staff grew large enough to allow the missionary doctors to take a day off each week, Jody and I would usually sleep in, have brunch, and then play Scrabble for a couple of hours. We would talk and talk while we did something we enjoyed. These days, I head for the kitchen as soon as I get home from work to help with supper and clean up, but more importantly to talk and debrief about our days.

If your spouse likes doing something special, create events at home or in the area—a picnic, a candlelight dinner for two with the kids sent elsewhere, a special movie night, etc. If she likes gifts, make them if you can't buy them or bring them back from trips. I almost always had a dozen roses in my hand when I returned from a trip to Nairobi. To my wife they said, "I was thinking of you and you are special."

Find something you and each child like to do together, and give them some special time with you do it. My kids liked stories and their favorite ones were the ones I made up. When they were younger, I had a continuing adventure story that serialized with them as I put each one to bed. I was involved in their hobbies and I involved them in mine. I wanted some special time with each of my children so they would feel special.

Minister as a Family
All of your family members are missionaries. The best way to avoid resentment or negative feelings is to look for group and individual ministry activities for you, your spouse, and your children. I especially did this while on the field. The kids could help the children in the pediatric ward by using puppets, taking pictures, bringing crayons for coloring, or telling a story. Form a family singing group if you have talent in this area. Take your family to services where you may be speaking. Have your children help write your prayer letter, prepare an article for your mission magazine, take pictures, or be in the video you are shooting. Teach them how to share Christ at the appropriate age. If you start early, it will come naturally later on.

I followed a different principle when the kids were school aged and we were on home assignment. I was very judicious about taking them on ministry trips during the school year. Studies show how important routines are in children's lives. We lived near family, Jody stayed home with the children, and I did not spend long periods on the road. I went to a mission conference and then came home for most of the week. We even tried to live in the same house during each deputation. I knew it was important to put down home country roots and help keep their lives more stable when they were facing the challenges of school, new friends, and fitting in. During school breaks, we would minister together more.

Play the Challenge Game
Studies show the best way to closely knit a family together in the U.S. is to go camping. Why? Because you face a common challenge together in the midst of a great adventure. Don't shield your children from personal and group challenges—perhaps it's a difficult trip, the need for support funding, or going to boarding school at the appropriate age for the specific child (everyone is different). When our children went to boarding school, it was much more difficult on us than it was on them. Sure, there were some tears at first, but soon they were having a ball. They couldn't wait to get back to sports, friends, events, and even studying after school breaks.

Our U.S. counterparts have to strategize how to give their children real challenges. Often on the mission field, you are surrounded with them. Use them to stretch your children, increase their dependency on God, and learn faith. Shielding children from challenges drains their spirit of adventure and innovation while taking the fun out of life. If you don't provide challenges for them, they will find their own in ways that may not be good.

Basic Training
You may have heard Dr. John Patrick's talk on, "Why Are There No Hittites on the Streets of New York?" The answer is that the Hittites did not teach their children their basic beliefs at home (Deuteronomy 11:19). It is easy to get so caught up in ministering to others that you forget your primary unreached people group, the earthly family God gave you. It is essential to have family devotions and prayer in an age appropriate manner. Just as important and crucial as it is to tell Bible stories, read Scripture, and pray, there is more to "basic training." It is telling your immediate and extended family's stories. This is crucial because you are separated from grandparents, uncles, and aunts on the field. Children need to know their story so they can see how they fit into the larger picture. As you paint that picture, keep it up to date. When children are young, use pictures and tapes. We used to make a tape to send home every week with the kids talking to their grand-

parents and other relatives. They would listen when we got a tape back. Missionary kids run a real risk if they are unattached, especially when they return to your home country for higher education. As they get older, work hard to facilitate relationships with cousins and other friends from your home country. Invite them out for a visit. Encourage letters or small gift giving. Send pictures. Basic biblical training and a family picture to fit into will build a firm foundation for your children when the storms of life arrive.

Celebration

Traditions and celebrations are important, especially when you are isolated. When our kids were young, there were not many missionary children their age on the compound, so we invited all of their "uncles" and "aunts" to their birthday parties. We started that tradition in residency with my oldest child Jason's first birthday. I was on call in my second year of residency so Jody baked a cake, got cone birthday hats and noise-makers, and brought it all with Jason in his stroller to the house staff call quarters. I still laugh when I see the picture of all the residents dressed in scrubs with their funny hats on and Jason with birthday cake smeared all over his face.

It is also important to maintain or start family traditions and get everyone involved in making them happen. One missionary family always had a Christmas evening drop-in party. As difficult and expensive as it was to get fireworks, I tried to have those available for July 4. We had Christmas ornaments for each child at Christmas to illustrate something important to them that year. If we couldn't buy them, we made them. Traditions are one of the glues binding families together. Whether it is a special food, "your" vacation spot, or the way you open the presents on Christmas morning, work hard to make special memories.

Worldview

Maximize your worldview experiences. I don't mean worldview in the sense of your basic beliefs or the lens you view the world through, but the unique opportunities you have to see the world. If anything, I wish I had done more of this type of family bonding. I know you don't have lots of money, but this is an area where you should save and skimp to take advantage of unique opportunities. Stop in foreign countries as you travel to and from your place of service or do unique things in your own region. One of the things I've kicked myself for was that I never took Jody on a hot air balloon ride across the Masaai Mara game preserve in Kenya. It cost $300 which was a great deal of money for a poor missionary in the 1980s. Truthfully, we had the savings to have made a memory we would never have forgotten. Our kids still talk about visiting France, seeing Germany, and going to museums in London, but there were many more things we could have done with a little creative planning and effort. Don't miss the educational and bonding opportunities around you.

Inquire Within
Educating your children may present unique challenges. Most mission organizations give wide latitude in paying for and giving parents discretion in how they educate their children. Even in a family, children's dispositions and needs may widely vary. One child may be an early adapter to boarding school while another one does much better in a homeschool environment. As I've dealt with missionary families and watched the process, I'm convinced the key is not where you educate your children, but how you inoculate a passion for inquiry, a passion for increasing knowledge. It is not so much who the teacher is, but how much the child wants to learn. The best parents model a love for learning and facilitate their children's everyday education through routine experiences. I remember a trip to the Kenyan coast where Jody started facilitating inquiry with questions. "Do you know what kind of fish are in the Indian Ocean? I don't. Why don't you find out and tell me?" Encyclopedias, books, and even questioning older missionaries who had been there were methods they used to find the answers. "What other animals live in the ocean?" "How far would we have to swim to get to India?" "What tribes live along the coast?" "What do they eat?"

Get the idea? The key to education is teaching children to educate themselves and always be inquisitive. It is giving them a love for books and teaching how to use them. It is making learning fun and giving them a sense of accomplishment so they teach themselves for a lifetime. Yes, they need to learn specific subjects, but I would focus on spending less time in the formal classroom and more time in a fascinating world learning those subjects. The goal should be less about grades and more about knowledge. Family does matter.

CHAPTER 33
SCHOOL DAZE

Our children's education almost kept us from going to the mission field. In 1980, every child in Kenya went to boarding school beginning in second grade at the young age of seven. We could not imagine that, so school became a recurrent topic of discussion during my last year of residency as we raised our support. Our oldest child Jason would be three years old when we arrived in Kenya, and seven did not seem that far away.

We began looking at our options. The homeschooling movement was just starting and Jody's sister was one of its pioneers. Jody pumped her for information and began looking at curriculums. Despite what she learned, she was not comfortable taking on the challenge since she wasn't trained in primary education. She was thrilled when she found out another new doctor's spouse, scheduled to arrive about the same time as us, was a primary teacher. They began to plan to open a small school for all our children and others.

I still remember discussing whether we should come home when the kids got to high school and then return when they went to college. Then God began to deal with our lack of faith. His still small voice said, "Dave and Jody, do you believe I can take care of everything EXCEPT your children? Do you think only you can assure their safety, their education, and their future?"

He reminded me how well the other missionary kids at Tenwek had turned out. When I went to Tenwek as a student in college, Dr. Steury's eight-year-old son took me on a tour of the compound and shared facts about the birds, fauna, and much more. I had been very impressed with his maturity and knowledge.

The question boiled down to this, "Can I really trust God?" It is a question every missionary has to deal with whether it is for issues of disease, personal safety, or education. And it is a question that doesn't disappear when you reach the mission field. God entrusted your children to you. You want to raise them to love the Lord and serve Him. You want them to be well-adjusted, mature, caring, deeply spiritual, highly educated, and much more.

The problem is that in the midst of seriously undertaking your important parenting responsibilities you can turn God's gift to you into your God.

It is not the first time that's happened. The first missionary God sent into a foreign country had the same problem.

The sadness and stress of infertility is much worse in many cultures than it is in the U.S. Where we served in Africa, the husband could send his new wife back to her home and demand his dowry back if she did not become pregnant within the first two years of marriage. If that happened, her life was over as far as she was concerned. Many women committed suicide when faced with this disgrace. If the husband didn't exercise his right of rejection, he came under intense community pressure to take a second wife so he could have children to continue his lineage.

I dealt with many desperate couples who came to the hospital begging me to help them conceive and spent many hours as a detective trying to figure out their problem and help them. Those couples who got pregnant after treatment experienced a joy that knew no bounds! I was their hero!

I was thinking about that recently while pondering the story of Abraham and Sarah. In their eyes, God inexplicably delayed fulfilling His promise to them. I suspect they doubted it would ever happen as the years and decades flew by. Out of their desperation, they tried surrogacy which led to a tragedy continuing today with Arabs hating Jews and Jews hating Arabs.

In His time, God did keep His promise. Reading between the lines, I imagine that their excitement and exhilaration knew no bounds.

Ancient Abraham probably acted like a lovesick newlywed, overprotecting Sarah during her pregnancy and ensuring she had the best midwife when his intensely desired son came into the world.

After that birth, his pride knew no bounds. The most important thing in his life was his son. He guarded him from injury, gave him the best education, and doted on him in every way. This was the child of his old age! There would be no other children and he loved him more than anything.

And that was the problem. He thought he had to do both God's job and his own. He thought all the details and responsibilities in raising Isaac depended on him. The entire burden was on his shoulders.

So one day God asked Abraham to put his son on the altar. It didn't make sense. Why would God give him Isaac and then ask him to kill his son like a sacrificial lamb? Even worse, his son was old enough to understand what was happening! How could he as a father look into his son's eyes and then plunge a knife into his heart? But as you hear on TV when the emergency broadcast system is activated, this was "only a test." God asked Abraham to demonstrate that he loved and trusted Him more than he loved his precious son.

This test is given to every missionary many times during his or her career. It is a test you have to pass:

- When you say yes to God's call.
- When you climb on the plane to head overseas for the first time with your children holding your hands.
- When you cry and hug your kids as they head off to boarding school.
- When you bring your teenagers back to the U.S. and say a tearful goodbye in front of their college dorms before you head back to the field.

God was right. We were not yet like Abraham. We had not put what we considered most precious, our children, on the altar. Through more prayer and reading God's Word, we made that commitment. That doesn't mean we unhooked our brains and common sense and abrogated our responsibilities to our children. We just operated from a different assumption, a foundation of trust and belief that God could guide us, that He was by our side, and that He had a plan all worked out. Let me share a few principles we learned in the process.

- Every child is different. What works for one, may not be the best option for another.
- Now more than ever, mission organizations do not want to dictate educational options to missionaries and are very open to funding the option you choose.
- The mission field can often provide a wonderful community for raising your children. Other missionaries and some nationals become "uncles" and "aunts" who are much closer to your children than their real uncles and aunts could ever be. Our children are adults with children of their own, but they still love and are close with their missionary "uncles" and "aunts."
- Missionary kids as a group are high achievers later in life. They are comfortable with different people and different cultures. They love to travel and have a much broader range of experiences than kids in their home country. They have a more realistic opinion of themselves and a biblical worldview. They have seen suffering, pain, and poverty, and genuinely care about people.
- They are not money focused. They have been rich (when they are with their overseas national friends) and they have been poor (compared to their friends on home assignment.)
- We did not lack educational tools. People were eager to help us educate our children well. In the mid-1980s when most school rooms in the U.S. did not even have a computer, our little one-room school had three computers for eight children. We also had the latest audio and video aids.
- Boarding schools can be poor, average, or great. Most are great like the one we had. We told the children they could go to boarding school when they were ready. The two oldest went in fifth and sixth grade. They missed us and we missed them, but we saw enormous spiritual, educational, and emotional growth in their lives during this time. They still consider their boarding school the best school they ever attended.
- Boarding school was much harder on us than it was the kids. If we were not careful, we could communicate that to them in our words, tone, and actions, thereby making the whole situ-

ation much more difficult. If we approached boarding school positively, they did too.

We utilized lots of different options. We homeschooled, had a one-room school house, and sent two of our kids to boarding school. God used every one of these options for our children's good during different phases of our service overseas.

When God called us back to the states, do you know what one of our biggest battles was? We did not want to bring our children back to the U.S. school system and culture. Doesn't God have a sense of humor? What we feared most was now what we valued most. We weren't dazed, confused, and unclear for very long. We just had to remind ourselves we had already put our children on the altar. God could take care of our children in the social and spiritual jungle of the states.

He did!

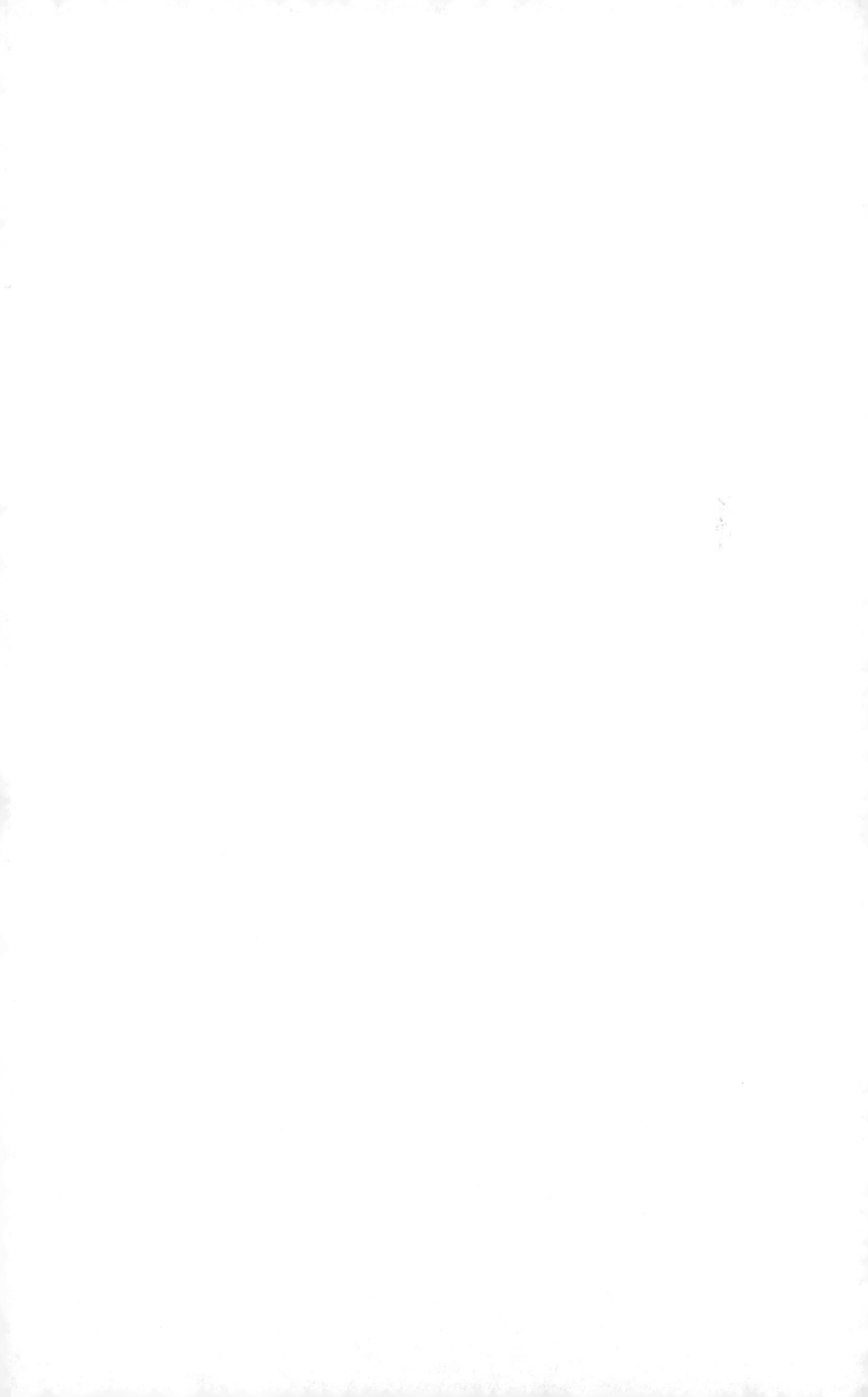

PART 10
PERSONAL AREAS

CHAPTER 34
SELF-CARE

Let's get personal. For long-term success in medical missions, you have to take care of yourself. Your life is a marathon, not a sprint, and you have to avoid injury and be in great condition to stay in the race.

Believe it or not, I was a runner in high school. I did best in the long distance events like 400 to 1,600 meters. It took discipline to start fast enough to get into a winning position, but not so fast that I wore out prematurely. Then I tried to get into a sustainable pace for the long haul, knowing I might need a final all-out-burst of effort if I was challenged at the end.

Life on the mission field is just like that. As a new missionary, you want to start strong and find your place in the relay team of your colleagues. You have to run to stay in the race until the end while being prepared for those times of extraordinary effort.

Your first step in good self-care is to evaluate where you are currently. This is true whether you are dreaming of working in missions, preparing for missions, just starting, or are well into your mission career. What are your strengths? What are your weaknesses in keeping your spiritual, emotional, physical, relational, family, and work life in balance?

I know I can get too absorbed in my work if I'm not careful. Emotionally, I stay on an even keel no matter how big the storm. I'm not prone to anxiety, worry, or depression. I enjoy people but don't have to be with them all of the time. I stay in fair shape but could benefit from a regular exercise program to increase my endurance. Spiritually, I have a regular devotional life and I'm active in my church. My wife Jody and I love being together and especially enjoy doing projects or traveling together. Get the idea?

One helpful point is to talk to your spouse or a close friend as you do this self-evaluation. The other person will see things you can't see for yourself. If it is hard to do it in person, offer a list of questions to answer on paper and encourage them to be frank. If your ego can take it, seeing yourself through someone else's eyes is very helpful.

An annual personal retreat is also beneficial. If you don't take one, you get so busy doing everyday tasks you don't take time to take your "wellbeing" pulse. Another way to do this is through a formal evaluation process with your supervisor. In a mission situation, that should include more than just how well you are doing your job and whether you are involved in spiritual outreach. It should be a 360 degree view of how you are doing on all fronts.

Each January, the President and President-elect of CMDA take me through that process. It starts with me doing a self-evaluation based on a detailed list of questions I pass on to them before we meet. We then sit down together with everything on the table, no questions barred. "What is my greatest source of frustration?" "Who rubs me the wrong way?" "How am I succeeding in my work and personal goals?" "What am I going to be working on in the next year?" and on and on.

We agree on a set of goals that I will report back on at the end of the next year. Those goals become a set of personal priorities. As you can imagine, this changes things. A couple of years ago, the board came back and said, "We are concerned you aren't taking your vacation. That is not healthy in the long run; from now on, taking vacation is not an option. We want you to take all of it and inform us when you have." Whoa! That changed my priorities. I finished the year feeling better than in a long time and had one of my most productive years.

Last year, they responded to my self-assessment that I felt my work was falling into a predictable pattern as CMDA matures and I missed the big challenges and new mountains to climb. That is what I thrive on. Together we made some plans to facilitate some new challenging initiatives personally and corporately.

Get the idea? Before you can decide where you need to grow, you first need to know where you are. Then put together a plan to grow holistically in every area of your life. Write it down. Share it with others, especially an accountability partner who can monitor your progress.

Okay, I hear your excuse, because I have used it myself. "Dave, you don't know how busy my life is. How overcommitted I already am. I can't add another thing."

Listen to yourself. You have just given the foundational reason for doing a self-assessment and making and keeping a plan. That doesn't mean doing more, but doing the most important things. It may mean doing less. You are never going to get to where you want to be unless you take some time to evaluate and plan.

I believe everyone needs to be a "Timothy" and have a "Timothy" in their lives—someone who is mentoring you and someone you are mentoring. When you are young, it is harder to find someone to mentor than to be mentored; as you get older, that equation inverts. Both activities are healthy for both parties.

A few years ago, I brought on a young pastor to serve as the Director of Church and Leadership Ministries at CMDA, knowing full well he was unlikely to be at CMDA more than two years. He showed great leadership and innovation everywhere he served. His next logical step was to lead a parachurch ministry, but I knew his capabilities would increase exponentially if he was mentored for a time before he took on this new role. There were a good number of areas critical to his success that he had little knowledge in.

We spent time together every week in a formal supervisory time, but learning flowed both ways. He was always watching how I handled a wide variety of situations and learning from my example. I kept stretching him with bigger assignments, especially in the areas he had the least knowledge or experience. Less than two years after he joined CMDA, he became president of a struggling parachurch ministry. He came off the blocks fast, positioned himself to win with a great race plan, and is now settling into a ground-eating pace. I still contact him often to get reports, offer advice, and provide encouragement. When I look at the last few years, I see this as one of my major "accomplishments" because it will bear enormous fruit in the lives of others. It was very good for me as well!

You need someone as a mentor or accountability partner to share your joys and frustrations with on a regular basis. Someone to whom you can reveal your innermost struggles. Someone who can pick you up, brush you off, and get you back into the race when you fall down or become exhausted. Someone who can pull you aside and frankly tell you, "You are running this race all wrong," and then advise you how to do better. One of the keys of self-care is having another person who deeply cares for you.

My accountability partner is my best friend and second-in-command here at CMDA. We share with each other things we wouldn't share with anyone other than our spouse. We encourage each other, provide a place to blow off steam, and tell each other when we need to slow down. We bounce our best ideas off each other and then sharpen them together. We care for each other's families and help each other out with whatever project we are doing at home or at work.

Of all the things that contribute to who I am and what I do in service to God, my accountability relationships have the largest impact and give me the greatest satisfaction. If you don't have someone like that in your life, look around and see who might fill that role. If there is no one in sight, begin to pray God will bring that person into your life.

CHAPTER 35
FORGIVENESS

I wish I knew then what I know now. I'll call her Mary. She was a mess. I saw her for the first time during my last year of residency and had to wade through a swamp of her psychosomatic complaints. She didn't complain about what was really wrong, but high blood pressure, depression, a cigarette addiction, and relationship difficulties with her husband were all dutifully noted on her problem list. And yet I sensed these were merely symptoms of a bigger issue, but I couldn't put my finger on it during a fifteen-minute visit.

I scheduled her back for a complete history and physical exam. She got evasive when I questioned her about her sexual history, but she finally let it spill out. Her stepfather sexually abused her when she was thirteen years old. It was like I had discovered a huge abscess—tense, throbbing, and full of puss—but I didn't know how to incise and drain it. I wrote prescriptions for her medical problems and referred her for counseling. I was more successful with hypertension medications than the counselor was with advice. Mary was chock full of bitterness and anger.

I realize now the real issue counseling didn't deal with was she wasn't willing to forgive her dead stepfather for what he did. Her lack of forgiveness was corrupting her marriage that now teetered on divorce. It was affecting her health through her nicotine addiction and aggravating her blood pressure. Her anger turned inward and was fueling her depression. She was hovering on the border of becoming suicidal.

Mary came to mind one day when I conducted an interview for *Christian Doctor's Digest* with psychologist Dr. Dick Tibbits on his book *For-*

give to Live. Like you, I memorized Ephesians 4:32 as a child, "And be ye kind one to another, tenderhearted, forgiving one another, even as God for Christ's sake hath forgiven you" (KJV).

Easy to say, hard to do.

Like Mary, I've struggled to forgive and let resentment eat at me like a cancer. No, I wasn't sexually assaulted, but there have been times I've considered myself abused or taken advantage of by others. Some were big issues with patterns of abuse and others were isolated incidents. Almost all of my discontent was perpetrated by other Christians. I can think of two people in particular who gave me sleepless nights that I spent praying and hoping God would give them what I thought they so richly deserved. I dreamed I would be justified and they would be punished. It took me a considerable amount of time to truly forgive them.

If you don't learn how to really forgive, I bet you have been there too. It is inevitable in the social pressure cooker of the mission field where you are unwillingly bound together with others in a high stress situation. Or perhaps you have an emotional abscess you've never fully dealt with from an event in your past which is affecting your emotional or mental health. Forgiveness is needed to incise the corruption. Until that is done, you can't proceed down the road to recovery. In his highly acclaimed book, Dr. Tibitts shares ten principles of forgiveness. My experience confirms their validity to me. He admits that true forgiveness is not easy, can take time, and involves a conscious decision.

He states that forgiveness begins when you:

1. Accept that life is not fair and that others may play by a different set of rules than you do. (Even other Christians you expect so much more from.)
2. Stop blaming others for your circumstances. (Everyone seems to want to be a victim these days to flee personal responsibility. "You've caused me to be this way.")
3. Understand that you cannot change the person who hurt you; you can only change yourself. (You are not God. Nor can you control God and make Him the instrument of your retribution.)

4. Acknowledge the anger and hurt that some unpleasant or even harmful event is causing you. (Admit to yourself where the real problem lies.)
5. Reframe your story of hurt—your "grievance story"—by placing the hurtful events in a broader context than your current point of view. (It is easy to focus on the grievance and not see it is just a smaller part of the whole picture of what God has done for you.)
6. Recognize that only you can make the choice to forgive. (It is what God expects but only you can do it through a willful decision.)
7. Shift your view of the offender by humbly choosing to empathize with his or her life situation. (The human desire is to demonize the offender instead of admitting that God loves and cares for the offender as much as He cares for you. That person is the victim of the devil's machinations and needs prayer, not condemnation.)
8. Intentionally move from discontent toward contentment. (Forgiveness is a matter of will.)
9. Understand that forgiveness will take time and cannot be rushed. (God can do it in an instant, but He usually teaches us to depend on Him as we go through the forgiveness process.)
10. Take responsibility for your life and your future. No more blame, "what ifs," or self-pity. I have free will and God's help, and He is bigger than this. He understands betrayal, hurt, and unfair treatment because He experienced it all Himself. He said, "Father, forgive them, for they know not what they do" (Luke 23:34, ESV).

If you want to live, at some point you must choose to forgive.

If this is an area where you are struggling, I recommend getting a copy of Dick Tibbits' book. It is two hundred pages and is full of practical steps and biblical principles that can bring comfort and healing.

Or God may want you to help others—a friend, family member, or patient. It is one of the most loving things you can do. Johann Lavater said it well, "He who has not forgiven an enemy has never yet tasted one of the most sublime enjoyments of life!"

CHAPTER 36
FLAMEOUT

On October 14, 2004, Pinnacle Flight 3701 crashed near Jefferson City, Missouri. While ferrying a 50-seat passenger plane from Little Rock, the pilots decided to see what the plane could do. They first did some acrobatic moves and then decided to climb at an excessive speed to 41,000 feet, far above the recommended maximum altitude. They overheated both engines in the attempt so they slowed the plane down to almost stall speed to cool the engines. The anti-stall system would have automatically forced them nose-down to take the plane to a safer altitude, but they overrode it four times, resulting in both engines flaming out. The plane plummeted.

They put the nose down to gain speed in an attempt to restart the engines, but the overheated turbine blades had expanded and the engines were jammed. They delayed notifying ground control of their plight for fourteen minutes during repeated failed attempts to restart their engines. By then, they had lost so much altitude they could not glide to an airport. They crashed two and a half miles from the end of the runway between two rows of houses in a ball of flames. Both of the pilots died.

Those pilots sound like some medical missionaries I know. Okay, I admit it, I was one of them. So instead of ragging on you, I will rag on me. You've heard me talk about how overwhelming the situation was when I first arrived at Tenwek and the need to start a nursing school. But I had been professionalized to believe that when the going gets tough, the tough get going. It was going to take extraordinary effort to carry my regular work load at the hospital while working to develop the nursing school at the same time. I went into a steep climb to take my work output to 41,000 feet.

I wrote funding proposals at night, worked on administrative issues on weekends, started new programs, designed buildings, recruited new missionaries, learned computer programming to design database systems, and even personally kept the accounts when we built our hydroelectric project. The ministry began to expand and develop. It began to change, but unfortunately, so did I.

Most of this happened in my second term when Dr. Steury was on home assignment in the U.S. I was in charge and thought, "I can push really hard this year while he is gone. I want him to see lots of improvements when he returns."

He didn't return on time. His routine physical found colon cancer. The operation went well, but he formed massive adhesions and obstructions that couldn't be released on repeated surgeries. They put in a TPN line and sent him home. I still remember the day I heard he was not coming back to Tenwek, probably forever.

My engines were overheating and the stress was evident. I was working every minute of every day and far into every night when I wasn't on call. I was getting irritable and pushing people more than leading them. I didn't have time for regular devotions or time with God. I thought, "Surely He understands. I'm doing all of this for Him. It's not my fault Ernie isn't here to help. I'm trapped, and the only way out is to just work harder and more efficiently doing all the work of a full-time doctor, a full-time administrator, and a full-time developer." Since my office was at home, I was near the kids and Jody but had little real time with them except at hurried meals. No kicking a soccer ball in the yard or a leisurely walk down to the river.

The stall indicator began to repetitively flash a warning, but I kept manually overriding it. My engines were running in the red. I was about to flame out, but two things kept me from crashing.

Jody summed it up pretty succinctly to me one day when she said, "You're not much fun to be with anymore." Increasingly, she felt she worked for me instead of being my wife—doing my laundry, making sure I had a meal no matter how late I was, and keeping the children out of my way. Her comment was like a flash of lightening in the darkness of my work obsession.

Secondly, miraculously, providently, God healed Dr. Steury. One day everything opened up and he could eat. He returned within a few months to share the load. I woke up and realized I had to put the nose down and get to a safer and sustainable flight altitude. That took discipline of a totally different sort. Now it's your turn.

As a medical missionary (or spouse), you are smart, hardworking, success-oriented, a problem solver, and more than a little obsessive compulsive. (Just the kind of doctor I want for my personal physician!)

The problem is those that great traits and talents are your greatest liabilities when exercised to the extreme. If the devil can't get you to ignore God's call, he will get you to work yourself to death. I've seen it again and again. Here is what I learned and now practice to avoid flaming out.

Set Margins
Be honest and recognize your boundaries in work, sleep, exercise, spiritual growth, and thriving relationships. Everyone is different. I need seven hours of sleep per night on average. You may get by with six. Step back from your limit by 5 or 10 percent to give you space to take opportunities that may arise.

At the same time, realize you may have to exceed those margins at times—perhaps another doctor gets sick or an epidemic fills your hospital to overflowing. You can exceed your limits for a period of time, but get down to a safer altitude inside your margins as soon as possible. Flameout happens when you go too hard for too long.

No Fly Zones
Create a culture of protected time. At Tenwek, our days off were sacrosanct when we finally instituted them. Since we lived where we worked, it was easy for someone to call or drop by our house to get advice on a problem. We badly needed to mentally leave our heavy work load when we physically could not do so. The standard was established that you didn't bother employees on their days off unless it was for purely social reasons. A day off truly became a real day off to restore, renew, and recharge. Of course, the other side of the equation had to work as well. No sneaking in some of your usual work.

Develop Habits and Traditions to Unplug
Jody and I developed the tradition of playing Scrabble for a couple of hours on my days off. In reality, it was a focused time for us to sit down and talk, catch up, and enjoy each other's company. Scrabble was the excuse. Find a hobby you enjoy which can absorb your mind. I got into carpentry, ham radio, and reading books. Other doctors collected stamps or gardened.

Today, I've designed and developed a beautiful English flower garden at our house. I nurture plants from seeds, add onto a drip irrigation system, and spend time in the garden with Jody pruning, weeding, and cutting our flowers. We put in a vine-covered gazebo with a little table where we can have lunch or supper and enjoy the beauty. I'm restored and renewed when I'm working in my garden.

Restoration Zones
Plan regular time to get away to relax. Don't do too much or go too far. Focus on relationships, lots of sleep, prayer, Bible study, good exercise, and doing the things you enjoy. These times are the built-in flameout prevention system. Use them.

Battery Charger
Your responsibilities are too big to tackle by yourself. Only Christ can give you peace amidst the stress, compassion among the masses, and joy in the midst of unrelenting demands. Every night I put my cell phone in its charger by my bed. If I forget and then use it a lot the next day, the screen goes dead. What makes us think our spiritual batteries won't die if we don't get charged up by God every day?

Find an Overseer
All of us need an accountability agent. Someone who sees us better than we see ourselves. Someone we will listen to and act upon their advice. Someone to say, "Slow down. You are pushing too hard." Or "Your life is getting out of balance. It is time to get back on course."

You can't run a marathon at sprint speeds. Learn to pace yourself and you will not only run the race well, but win. God will be glorified. You will be fulfilled. Others will be blessed.

CHAPTER 37
POINTS ON TIME

Don't complain you don't have enough time. You have the same amount of time each day as Albert Einstein, Mother Teresa, and Michelangelo. The issue is not lack of time, but how you are investing the time you have each day. Thomas Jefferson advocated, "Determine never to be idle. No person will have occasion to complain of the want of time who never loses any. It is wonderful how much can be done if we are always doing."

Don't misinterpret Jefferson's words. He was not advocating working twenty-four hours a day, but instead was supporting investing your time in what is important.

The topic of time management recently came up when I had some problems with my computer calendar program. My son was trying to help me repair the problem and noticed how many events I had each day such as supervision meetings, media interviews, writing projects, strategic phone calls, and speaking engagements. It was a teachable moment as I shared something I had learned about investing my time well.

If you are like most missionaries, it seems as though there is not enough time in a day for all you have to do, much less what you want to do. I can relate to that. Please don't think I have it all together and always manage my time well. At the same time, I accomplish more than most people by employing the following principles.

Change Your Mind
Oftentimes, being busy is what we do to ourselves, not what life does to us. Some things are beyond your control. If you are faced with a

malaria epidemic, your time is not your own. Yet good time management is even more important during a crisis than during a normal period. Occasionally step back and use an objective to evaluate and answer the question, "How am I using my time?" If you are not investing your time well, change your mind. Make a conscious decision to apply good time management principles to your life and then act on them. Assessing how you are doing is critical to investing your time well.

Opt for Organization
Lack of organization robs you of time. Yesterday, it rained. I could have spent a number of minutes looking for my umbrella but organization solved that problem. The umbrella rack is right beside the front door where I head out to work. When I come home, that is where it goes so I can easily grab it on my way out the door. Multiply these few minutes by the dozens of things you do each day—looking for your keys, trying to locate your cell phone, or finding a pen—that can take less time if you get organized.

I travel a great deal so I have packing down to a science. I have two sets of toiletries. One is in my travel kit ready to grab and stick in my bag. I'm not looking for bits and pieces or constantly transferring items back and forth with each trip. I keep my suitcase in my closet instead of the attic so it is easy to grab. I have a mental checklist of what I need to take and can pack for a weekend trip in ten minutes. Whatever you have to do each day, how can you minimize the time wasted through good organization?

Clutter is the enemy of organization. Ruthlessly give away or donate things not needed. If you haven't used something in a year, you probably don't need it. Put things that you use often in easily accessible locations and file everything else away. Mark storage boxes with their contents so you can easily find items. I don't sort through drawers and cupboards looking for things in my workshop. Everything has its place on pegboards on my wall where I can find it at a glance and put it back where it belongs. I have a three-ring binder in my top right desk drawer containing reference lists I consult frequently. There are hundreds of things you can do to get organized. Get a good book on this subject and apply it. Opt for good organization. It will save you a ton of time.

Rally to Routines
I have daily, weekly, monthly, quarterly, and annual routines I keep on my computer calendar. For example, I avoid many time-robbing interruptions because I meet individually with every staff member I supervise at the same time every week. It gives me a chance to find out what is going on in their departments and what problems I can help solve. I can assign a new task, give encouragement and feedback, and set priorities.

At our board meetings each year, we have a number of routine subjects we assign to each meeting during the year. One meeting reviews the audit, examines our insurance policies, and reviews the staff policy manual. Another one sets budgets, nominates new officers, and does other routine tasks. We don't forget to do something because they are on the annual calendar. It also allows us to stagger tasks so we don't have too much work to do at any particular meeting. It creates a routine.

The added blessing is these routines don't take as much mental energy because they are good for us psychologically and physically. You can do simple routines while occupying your mind with more important things.

Be a Goaltender
Take time to list daily, weekly, monthly, yearly, and even lifetime goals. The Bible says, "Where there is no vision, the people perish…" (Proverbs 29:18, KJV). You need a vision for what you want to accomplish, what new skills you want to acquire, people you want to keep in contact with, and projects you want to accomplish. They can be specific or general goals. You may have a general goal of spending quality time with your family and a specific goal of reading through the Bible in a year.

Goals are meaningless unless they are connected to a measurable objective and a due date. What is the goal line you are trying to reach and when do you want to get there? I like to work backward from when I want to have big goals accomplished to figure out what I need to be doing now to accomplish them. In other words, big goals get broken into measurable milestones so I can see how I am progressing. I find checklists a great way to monitor my progress.

Pick Your Priorities

Once you have your goals, schedule them according to importance. It may make sense to get some small tasks out of the way so you can handle a big one, but at other times you need to block time out for a bigger task and ignore smaller goals so you can get the big item accomplished. Sometimes I put a sign on my door, "If it is an emergency, come in. If not, check back later. I'm focused on a project." It may be a presentation, an article to write, or a sermon to prepare. I've learned interruptions stifle the concentrated creativity needed for some things and I need to prioritize them and block out time. I've also learned some tasks are better done at different times of the day. I think and sound better on audio projects if I do them early in the day. By the end of the day, I do not sound so energized. Menial tasks like doing an expense report can be accomplished late in the day when my energy has dropped.

One of the most common time management mistakes is to focus on the urgent to the detriment of strategic goals that move your life or ministry forward. Prioritizing your goals and scheduling time to work on strategic items makes a big difference.

Sole Search

There are certain things others can do and certain things they cannot do. Understanding that, it is important to do only what you can do first. I can get tripped up spending too much of my time on things others can do as well or better while neglecting what only I can or must do. Visiting staff cannot run your healthcare ministry, create new programs, or develop management systems. However, they can see patients and free you up for the tasks that strategically move you forward.

Sometimes you need to train others to pick up things they can learn to do to help you out. Search out the things that only you can do. They are the most important things to focus your time on.

No Way

The more successful you are, the more people will ask you to do. They will want you on their board, committee, or advisory group. They will want you to speak, share your insights, or consult on a patient. The real skill is analyzing what you should or shouldn't do and then learn how to say, "No." People won't accept the excuse that you don't have time, but they can't argue with, "That unfortunately doesn't fit into my priorities right now." Another strategy to employ is to suggest someone else you think can accomplish the task. Of course, you should ask permission to suggest their name if you want to keep your friends!

It's possible that you may need someone to protect you from undue pressure to do more. That person may be your spouse who you have made a commitment to be at home with more or your supervisor. For example, I asked the CMDA board to establish a parameter stating I could not serve on other institutional boards without permission. It is now easy for me to say no to requests I don't really want to take because the board provides protection for me. I can focus my time on critical goals and priorities.

Time Tracking
Every once in a while, it is worth it to keep a detailed log of how you are spending your time. It is like counting calories. You may think you are staying on your diet, but you find out you really are not when you examine your diet diary. A time log reveals the truth of what is really going on. One of my time logs revealed I was spending way too much time on e-mail each day. I began dictating more and kept my answers shorter. I set a time in the morning I wanted to have my e-mail done and worked toward that goal. I picked up the phone more often since it took less time. I would have wasted lots of precious time if I hadn't identified this problem through time tracking.

Flex Time
Some tasks are going to take longer than expected so you need to build margin into your schedule. This flex time can be used to get ahead on menial tasks or devote to long-term projects if needed. It also improves your chances of completing all your goals on time while decreasing your stress. In addition, it gives you time for interruptions, divine appointments, and to minister to people when operations arise.

Sometimes the unexpected exceeds your flex time. That is when it is important to be flexible and extend your deadlines or find another solution. My schedule allows thirty minutes for supervisory meetings, but one particular meeting was consistently lasting fifteen minutes longer because their area of responsibility was complex. I had to flex and make that appointment 45 minutes and help that person be more organized so we could accomplish everything in that length of time.

Get Down
All of us need time to relax, refuel, and restore. You need down time. Don't forget to schedule time for fun and laughter. Spend time doing your hobby or visiting friends. Exercise and get adequate sleep so you can function at your best. These and other activities restore your energy and creativity while allowing you to live a balanced life. They also help you use your time efficiently. When you are tired or anxious, your creative juices don't flow and many tasks take twice as long to do.

I could add more principles, but these should get you started improving your time usage. Peter Drucker said it well, "Until we can manage time, we can manage nothing else."

I love improving my time management because it has instant awards. I have more time for hobbies, recreation, and relationships. Most importantly, I can make a greater difference in ministry and individual lives because I have been a good steward of God's gift of time to me. I don't want to spend time. I want to invest it. Don't you?

CHAPTER 38
CACHINNATION

Woody Allen certainly isn't a medical missionary, but he articulated the sentiments of many missionaries when it comes to fun: "Most of the time I don't have much fun. The rest of the time I don't have any fun at all."

Missionaries' days are long breathless sprints trying to catch up to an overwhelming workload. Nights are often spent in the operating room. When you add to those burdens—administration, management, communicating with supporters, spiritual ministry, and trying to have family time—fun falls off the curve. Fun and laughter are relegated to happenstance or more likely don't happen at all.

What do I mean by fun? I'm not talking about finding time to watch a video or even read a good book. Both are important breaks from your busy schedule, but what I'm talking about is putting more laughter into every day and planning times for cachinnation (to laugh loudly or immoderately). You know, the type of belly laughing and good times that you are going to be talking about for months.

Hey, it is a holy thing to laugh! The Bible says so. Remember the story of Sarah's infertility? God came to Abraham and told him Sarah would have a baby and he should be named Isaac which literally means "laughter." Why? Because Sarah first laughed in derision that God could give her a son with this old man, but then she laughed with joy after Isaac was born. In Genesis 21:6, Sarah said, "God has blessed me with laughter and all who get the news will laugh with me!" (MSG).

When God used Esther to save her people, the Jews created a new holiday for laughter (Esther 8:16, 9:17). David said, "…I'm whistling, laughing, and jumping for joy; I'm singing your song, High God" (Psalm 9:2, MSG). Ecclesiastes 3:4 reminds us there is "...a right time to cry and another to laugh" (MSG). David tells us how to give thanksgiving to God, "Bring a gift of laughter, sing yourselves into his presence" (Psalm 100:2, MSG). In Romans 12:15, we are told to, "Laugh with your happy friends when they're happy" (MSG).

Science demonstrates what the Bible already tells us is true. Dr. Lee Berk and Dr. Stanley Tan of California's Loma Linda University studied the effects of laughter and found it reduces blood pressure, decreases stress hormones, increases muscle flexion, and boosts immune function by raising the levels of T-cells, B-cells, and gamma interferon. It also causes the release of endorphins to reduce pain levels and produces a general sense of well-being. Other studies show increases in IgA, IgB, and complement with those levels remaining elevated for long periods of time.

Laughter is a good vitamin for the soul. You feel better and are healthier when you laugh. If you could package the effects of laughter into a pill, you would become wealthy overnight! Don't you love being around truly funny people? They make you feel good. Well, each of us can bring some laughter to others. The best way is to poke fun at yourself and what you do. Secondly, look for a source of laughter in common everyday occurrences and "crack a joke" about it. Take some time to read some jokes or funny stories and share them with others.

Have fun with your family. Before he passed away, Jody's dad had advanced Alzheimer's and lived with us. He had a rich life of ministry as a college professor, gymnastic coach, and mayor of his small town. Near the end of his life, he had trouble reading and his memory was largely gone, but he made me laugh because laughing is contagious. He loved watching "The Three Stooges" and did he cachinnate! His belly laughs were contagious and before I knew it, I was laughing too!

Find things to make your family laugh. We laughed a great deal with our family during a recent Christmas break. We shared funny stories from the past, told jokes, and played games. We learned one game you can play anywhere with a group of friends as long as you have paper and pens. Cut the paper into two-inch squares. Give each person as many pieces of paper as you have people in your group. You start by writing any word or phrase on your paper such as "mid-life crisis," "War and Peace," and "A Few Good Men." You have sixty seconds. You pass the paper to the person on your left who then has three minutes to draw that phrase without using words or numbers. Then they pass it to the person on their left. That person tries to decipher it and writes what they think the phrase is on another piece of paper. You keep up the sequence until it gets back to you. Then each person shares the results with everyone in the group. It is hilarious! For us, "A Few Good Men" ended up being Christopher Columbus discovering America!

It is also good to have periodic planned times for fun and games. If not, you will get consumed by everyday tasks. When we arrived on the mission field, we had "game night" every Friday evening with the other missionaries. We met at someone's house, had snacks, played games, did skits, and laughed so much. I still remember a game night when we all came dressed for Christmas. Have you ever seen a tropical Santa? I came in a baby blue leisure suit with a huge pillow that shook like a "bowl full of jelly" and a beard made out of a surgical mask and cotton balls. I had written an adaptation of "The Twelve Days of Christmas" to go with it. That was twenty-five years ago and I can still hear our laughter!

God tells us to laugh and it is good for us! What can you do to get more laughter in your life and the lives of your friends and colleagues? As you do, you will find the added benefit of better morale, better bonding, and better strength for what God calls you to do.

Here are a few funny quotes to get you started:

- "I didn't attend the funeral, but I sent a nice letter saying that I approved of it." – Mark Twain
- "They say such nice things about people at their funerals that it makes me sad to realize that I'm going to miss mine by just a few days." – Garrison Keillor
- "Skiing combines outdoor fun with knocking down trees with your face." – Dave Barry
- "No matter how rich you become, how famous or powerful, when you die the size of your funeral will still pretty much depend on the weather." – Michael Pritchard

CHAPTER 39
LEAVING WITHOUT LEAVING

Aren't vacations great! I recently returned from a week off, and I returned restored and renewed to a very busy schedule. Most people want to get away and travel when they have time off. You know, "vacation." I had a different goal since I travel all the time. I structured my time off as a "stay-cation." We stayed at home and Jody and I did some projects around the house, went to a couple of movies, took long walks, and read some books. My brother even came to visit for a few days and we went fly-fishing. One of the best trout fishing rivers in the U.S. is a few miles from my house. We had a banner fishing day as we floated the South Holston River and fished with small nymphs. They were so small you almost needed a magnifying glass to thread them on a three-pound test tippet line.

To be honest, this vacation was long overdue. I spent too many weeks in the office and too many weekends on the road since the beginning of the year.

Knowing a missionary's life, I know you need restoration even more than I do. You are likely in a remote situation where it is difficult and expensive to get away. The demands of providing healthcare are unrelenting. You have to work very hard to grab even a few moments for yourself.

I remember those days well. We usually got away for a couple of weeks each year to go to the beach with the kids. It was a two-day trip to get there and two-days back. We have wonderful memories of those times together. But those trips were totally inadequate to restore my emotional and mental batteries for an entire year. There had to be something else to do that on a regular basis.

I dubbed that "leaving without leaving" and I'm a great believer in it. As a missionary, you need outlets that restore and renew you personally. Of course, the most important thing is staying in God's Word and taking time for prayer and fellowship. Only God can provide the strength and wisdom for the challenges you face each day (and night!).

But "leaving without leaving" adds another indispensable dimension. I had to learn to disconnect and mentally leave when my body couldn't physically leave. I got onto this as I watched the other career doctors who had been on the field for years cope.

Dr. Steury was raised on a farm, so he loved growing a garden, raising chickens, and even keeping a herd of pigs who were fed leftovers from the hospital kitchen. Ernie would frequently transport fifty one-day-old chicks all the way from Nairobi when he was there on business. He created a "brooder" area in his basement where he kept the chicks warm with kerosene lanterns until he could transfer them to his chicken coop and grow them into tasty meals for all of us. He even injected a few of them with hormones so we could have some hens as big as "turkeys" for Thanksgiving. When he was working on his garden or dealing with his animals, he was "gone" because he was totally focused on what he was doing.

I enjoy a good mystery, thriller, or adventure story. Before we had a hydro plant, my routine was to climb into bed as soon as the lights blinked at 9 p.m. When the lights went out five minutes later, I would turn on our battery light and spend an hour or two totally disconnected from the challenges of everyday life. On Saturday evenings, I would crank up my ham radio and talk to other amateur radio operators from all over the world. There were fewer than 50 "hams" in Kenya, so as soon as I gave my call sign, everyone with a shortwave transmitter wanted to talk to me so they could add Kenya to their country list.

When I had a day off, you might find me down with my tools in my workshop making bookshelves or helping the kids with a project. Jody loved to sew so I built her a combination desk and sewing table.

When the days of videotapes arrived, we had a wonderful friend who taped movies and major sporting events and send them out by the box with work teams. Our house became the "Blockbuster" outlet at Tenwek. We had so many movies I created a database so other missionaries could come by and check them out of our "movie closet" to enjoy.

In some places, it is easier to mentally get away than it used to be. The internet, DVDs, Skype, and other outlets make it easier to "leave without leaving," but it is no less important. Let me share a few principles I learned on how to do it well.

Disconnect but Don't Escape
Watching a good movie or reading a book are great ways to disconnect when done in moderation. However, those pursuits lose their effectiveness if you do them all the time as an escape. A reasonable time away is refreshing, but spending all your free time trying to live in another world is an addiction.

Be Productive
The best hobbies and activities are those that produce something of value upon their completion—new relationships, something you have grown or built, or something to share with others. These days, I grow flowers in my cottage garden with Jody. It is refreshing to spend time together creating beauty we can share. Dr. Rudd makes wooden bowls to give away. He calls it "sawdust therapy" and is always eager to teach someone else.

Involve Your Loved Ones As You Can
Every hobby doesn't have to be done together but all of them should not be done apart, especially when they take significant time. Resentment is built in a marriage or family if anything steals time that rightfully should be theirs.

Make Sure Your Spouse Has an Outlet
If you are married, make sure to give permission and encourage your spouse to have a hobby or outlet they love. Your marriage will be better for it. Jody loved bird watching as we had more than one hundred species on our compound and more than seven hundred in Kenya. Occasionally I would go with her as she made her way around the area with binoculars and bird book in hand.

There are Seasons for Everything

I have a friend who is a great golfer. When he started having children, he gave up his hobby because it took too much time away from his family. He instead developed other hobbies he enjoyed and could do with his kids at home. Now that his children are grown, he is getting back into golf with his wife's blessing.

I had to learn this life-sustaining skill. I'm a very focused and goal oriented person; without periods of restoration or renewal, I found that my world was changing me. I reminded myself that even God took a day of rest, and I'm not God.

Maybe you are facing the same battle. If so, it is time to step back, do a checkup on your life, and reprioritize your schedule to make sure you make time to leave without leaving! You and those you love and serve will be better for it!

CHAPTER 40
WEALTH MANAGEMENT

I worked with one of the richest doctors in the world. On a daily basis, I watched him add to his net assets. The wonder of it was that he freely taught me his secrets to being extremely wealthy. I thought it only appropriate I share those secrets with you.

Before I do, you should know I think money is a good thing—if taken in the proper doses. Of course, too much or too little of it can be dangerous to your mental and even physical health. Have you noticed, no matter how much money we have, it never seems to be enough? It also doesn't bring contentment or happiness. People seem to be either anxious about getting more or fretting and worrying about losing what they have. Just listen to the discussions in the doctor's lounge!

Sure, money can buy lots of things—cars, vacation homes, expensive jewelry, beautiful knick knacks—but Frank Lloyd Wright revealed the dark side of that coin when he said, "Many wealthy people are little more than janitors of their possessions."

All the same, you and I should be good stewards of our money. We should manage it well. It enables us to take care of our families, pay our staff, and even retire some day from our hectic lives.

But I digress. Let me share with you what one of the richest doctors in the world taught and showed me about being wealthy.

First, I should never mistake money for riches. He taught me how to measure real wealth. He said the real measure of my wealth is how much I would be worth if I lost all my money. The real measure of my wealth is how much others value me for who I am, not for what I have in my bank account. He said my real wealth could be measured by the things money can't buy—love, relationships, respect, and contentment.

Secondly, if I want to be really wealthy, I need to keep my priorities straight. If I allow money to become my god, it will be my master and I will be its slave. Thus, I need to continually work to be the master of my money or money could easily become the master of me.

Thirdly, I need to learn to invest well to receive greater long-term returns. But his lessons on investments didn't focus on arbitrage, options, or cost averaging. He focused solely on high yield investments. He showed me the highest yielding investment I could make was to invest in the lives of others. He told me it didn't take special skills or abilities, just time. He would say, "Let those that you want to influence spend time with you. Ask them questions and have them query you. Not only will it help them to become all they are designed to be, but you will grow from it as well." He invested like that in me and it changed my life! As I worked with him daily, I found that net assets are built through kind words and deeds generously given every day to others. Thoreau was right, "Goodness is the only investment that never fails."

One last lesson he taught me in regards to money was generosity. John Wesley said, "When I have money, I get rid of it quickly, lest it find a way into my heart." Money can do that, especially if you consider it your most precious asset. As busy healthcare professionals, our "most precious" asset is not money, but time. And time is something you and I treasure the most because we have so little of it we can truly call our own. Yet, true generosity is not just a check you write each month or the handful of coins you drop in the Salvation Army bucket. True generosity is giving what you value most to others.

With these lessons in mind, he was the richest doctor I've ever known. Yet, he didn't own a house or a car until after he retired. When he finished his internship, he traveled to a remote corner of Africa to become the first doctor at a small bush clinic. For the first ten years, he was the lone doctor at the clinic, taking calls both day and night. On his short home assignments to the U.S., he raised money to buy equipment and build buildings. Others finally came to help him on both a short-term and a long-term basis. National staff was trained. Today, that hospital is a 280-bed tertiary care hospital surrounding the two small stone buildings that housed the original clinic. Its residency programs train some of the best family doctors and surgeons in the country. Recently, the hospital's nursing school was one of six out of forty-four schools in the country to have all of its graduates pass their exams, and it had one of the top two graduates in the country.

As wonderful as the facilities, programs, and services now are at Tenwek, that wasn't my teacher's most enduring legacy. His heritage bears higher dividends than that. To see it, you would have to see the lives of the nationals and expatriates he worked with and the lives of those he influenced with his character, word, and deeds. Dr. Steury's riches continue to grow and cultivate as those people he guided now influence others.

Now that is real wealth management!

FINAL THOUGHTS

One of the things I miss most about being a medical missionary is that I no longer have the opportunity to exercise my faith as much. There's no question that spiritual exercise has greater benefit than physical exercise. As missionaries, we depended on God and spiritually exercised on a daily basis. We prayed before we left for a clinic trip and let someone know when we should be back. If the car broke down somewhere out in the bush, we prayed that someone would come by to help us before the day was over. If not, we trusted someone from the hospital would come looking for us in the dark.

We prayed for every surgical patient before we picked up a scalpel. We prayed for more supplies when we were running short. We prayed that the seriously sick would receive healing, that the generator would come back on, that we would be able to fix a broken piece of essential equipment, and that God would protect our children at boarding school. We prayed for the staff and the funds we needed to improve our infrastructure and programs. We prayed all the time, trusted God, and saw His hand at work. Our spiritual muscles were strengthened by every faith exercise we undertook. We saw God working every single day.

As you read the huge variety of things that you might be called upon to do as a medical missionary, it may seem overwhelming. You may feel you don't have the aptitude, abilities, or experience to do many of them. I understand. I've felt that way as well many times. I could relate many stories where I felt I failed or at least didn't do a job as well as I hoped.

That reminds me of a couple of lines I wrote in my book *Leadership Proverbs*: "If you can't do something superbly, do it poorly until you get better at it. Experts weren't born that way."

Remember when you put in your first IV or did some other new thing? If I remember right, I had to stick my first patient three times...and he had great veins! Before long though, I could slip one in while half asleep. I became an expert through trial and error.

One of the greatest problems we have is limiting what God can do in and through us because we make excuses for not even trying. We refuse to exercise our faith. Remember, God is not expecting you to be successful. He is expecting you to be willing, teachable, and trusting. He wants you to go beyond your comfort zone and then rest in Him. To do otherwise out of fear of failure is often rooted in pride.

The other thing that holds us back is simply slothfulness. I know you are a hard worker, but our attitude when facing a unfamiliar challenge on the mission field is often to say we are too busy or something else is more important. I remember a hospital with close to ten physicians, but all of them refused to take the leadership role of being the medical superintendent. Without exception, they claimed they needed to spend more time with their families. The hospital was floundering.

Do you think it was God's design that there were no leaders? Of course not! God's Word is full of stories from cover to cover of the leaders He called to step up and face very difficult situations. It is easy to make excuses when we should be asking God, "Do you want me?" or "How can I serve you in this situation?"

If we do follow His direction, He fills in our voids. He takes us by the hand and says, "Yes, I know you don't know how to do what needs to be done, but I do. Trust me. Learn. Let's go on a faith adventure together. Not only will we get this done, but we will grow closer together as you lean more on me." When we are willing to seek His guidance, step out in faith, and trust Him, He does extraordinary things above our wildest dreams.

I know it will take personal sacrifice. Things worth doing always do. Throughout this book, you've seen the struggles I faced when I was appointed the leader of Tenwek Hospital. We didn't have clean water, twenty-four hour electricity, adequate staff, proper sewage, a pharmacist, good financial controls, adequate financial reserves, or good governance (and that is just the short list). I realized it was going to take extraordinary effort and sacrifice to get out of the deep ditch we were in. I was going to attempt to bring about so many changes while working full-time at the hospital and taking night call every three to four nights. I didn't know enough, I didn't have enough time, and I had little limited experience.

God reminded me that I just needed to volunteer, depend on Him, work diligently, and then see Him work. It was a miracle what He did over the next six years! It was so obviously not me, but Him who accomplished the miraculous. The joy was that He took me along as He accomplished His purpose.

I challenge you to take what you have learned in this book and ask God what He wants you to do with it. If you are still in preparation, don't forget to pack this book when you head to your place of service. If you are already serving, what needs to be tackled to make your healthcare outreach what He wants it to be? How does God want you to exercise your faith? What is the first step you should take to reach the goals and objective He has revealed? Take it and then take another step. Pray, believe, persist, and mobilize others.

The great 18th century missionary William Carey summed it up well, "Expect great things of God, attempt great things for God."

Then when you see God work, don't forget to fall down on your knees and thank Him for what He has done and for letting you be a part of it.

APPENDIX

About the Author

David Stevens, MD, MA (Ethics), serves as the Chief Executive Officer for the Christian Medical & Dental Associations. From 1981 to 1991, Dr. Stevens served as a missionary doctor in Kenya helping to transform Tenwek Hospital into one of the premier mission healthcare facilities in the world. Subsequently, he served as the Director of World Medical Mission, the medical arm of Samaritan's Purse, assisting mission hospitals and leading medical relief teams into war and disaster zones. As a leading spokesman for Christian doctors in America, Dr. Stevens has conducted hundreds of television, radio, and print media interviews. Dr. Stevens holds degrees from Asbury University, is an AOA graduate from the University of Louisville School of Medicine, and is board certified in family practice. He earned a master's degree in bioethics from Trinity International University in 2002.

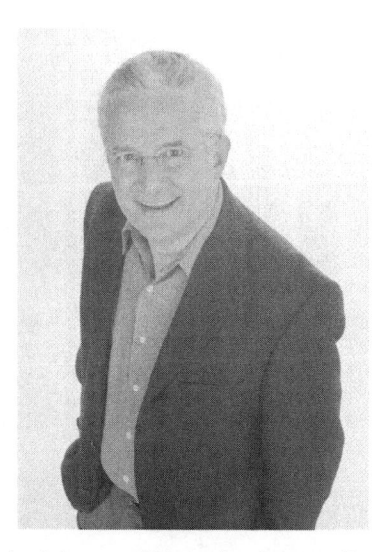

Dr. Stevens' experiences provide rich illustrations for inspirational and educational presentations at seminars, medical schools, conferences, and churches. His topics include stem cell research, human cloning, genetics, faith and health, physician-assisted suicide, international and community-based healthcare, emergency medical relief, abortion, and other medically related subjects. He is the author of *Jesus, MD*, co-author of *Leadership Proverbs*, and a regular contributor for *East Tennessee Medical News*.

About CMDA

The Christian Medical & Dental Associations was founded in 1931 and currently serves more than 16,000 members; coordinates a network of Christian doctors for personal and professional growth; sponsors student ministries in medical and dental schools; conducts overseas healthcare projects for underserved populations; addresses policies on healthcare, medical ethics, and bioethical and human rights issues; distributes educational and inspirational resources; provides missionary doctors with continuing education resources; and conducts international academic exchange programs. For more information about CMDA, visit *www.cmda.org* or call 888-230-2637.

CMDA's Mission Outreaches

CMDA is dedicated to domestic and international missions and has several mission outreach ministries. Its various ministries provide opportunities for healthcare professionals to use their God-given skills to meet the needs of others and share the gospel with them.

Center for Medical Missions – *www.cmda.org/cmm*
A program designed to serve domestic and international healthcare missionaries in their work as well as aid in the recruitment and retention of career medical missionaries. CMM also assists students with scholarships and overseas rotations.

Continuing Medical & Dental Education – *www.cmda.org/cmde*
A program designed to provide continuing education in a compact, multiple track model enabling medical and dental professionals serving overseas to affordably earn credit to assist in maintaining licensure in the U.S.

Global Health Outreach – *www.cmda.org/gho*
A short-term missions program that sends 40 to 50 medical, dental, and surgical outreach teams around the world. GHO disciples participants, grows national churches, shares the gospel, and provides care to the poor and needy.

Global Health Relief – *www.cmda.org/ghr*
An outreach ministry partnering with the Salvation Army for short-term relief work by showing the love and compassion of Christ to those affected by disasters around the world through medical, dental, spiritual, and psychological care and support.

Medical Education International – *www.cmda.org/mei*
A short-term missions program that sends healthcare professionals to teach in academic or clinical settings to bring transformation by advancing medical, dental, bioethical, and educational knowledge while sharing the gospel.

Pan-African Academy of Christian Surgeons – *www.cmda.org/paacs*
A commission that trains and disciples African surgeons to glorify God and provide excellent, compassionate care to those most in need. Training is offered at several well-established evangelical mission hospitals in Africa.

Recommended Mission Outreaches

Christ Community Health Fellowship – *www.cchf.org*
A community of Christian healthcare professionals who are committed to living out the gospel through healthcare among the poor. About half of the people who make up the CCHF community work in secular settings—community health clinics, universities, residency programs, etc. The rest of the CCHF community works in faith-based clinics that strive to provide distinctively Christian care.

Christian Pharmacy Fellowship - *www.cpfi.org*
A worldwide ministry of individuals working in all areas of pharmaceutical service and practice. Its mission is to serve Christ and the world through pharmacy.

Christian Physical Therapists International – *www.cpti.org*
An association of Christian physical therapists dedicated to encouraging, instructing, and challenging members in the physical therapy field to a deeper, more fulfilling walk with the Savior, equipping them to impact the lives of others with the gospel.

Fellowship of Christian Physician Assistants – *www.fcpa.net*
An organization intended to serve and represent Christian physician assistants and students. It provides members with mission service opportunities to network and share fellowship with others.

MAP International – *www.map.org*
A Christian health organization that partners with people living in conditions of poverty to save lives and develop healthier families and communities. It responds to the needs of those it serves by providing medicines, preventing disease, and promoting health to create real hope and lasting change.

medicalmissions.com – *www.medicalmissions.com*
The largest gathering of medical missions professionals and students in the world. Learn about medical mission trips, opportunities for doctors and nurses, and find out about upcoming conferences focused on healthcare missions. A ministry of Southeast Christian Church, it hosts the annual Global Missions Health Conference in Louisville, Kentucky.

Recommended Mission Outreaches

MedSend – *www.medsend.org*
A ministry enabling healthcare professionals to serve spiritually and physically needy people around the world in the name of Christ by making their monthly educational loan payments while they serve. Since being founded in 1992, MedSend has approved educational loan repayment grants to almost 500 healthcare professionals serving around the world.

Nursing Christian Fellowship - *www.ncf-jcn.org*
A ministry of and for nurses and nursing students. NCF provides a local, regional, national, and international network to bring the message of Jesus Christ and a Christian worldview to nursing education and practice. NCF provides Christ-centered resources and programs that equip nurses and students for ministry in nursing, including spiritual care, ethics, and a Christian perspective on nursing issues.

World Medical Mission – *www.samaritanspurse.org*
The medical arm of Samaritan's Purse, World Medical Mission was established in 1977 to assist general surgeons who wanted to volunteer for short-term mission trips. Today, they place volunteer Christian physicians, dentists, and other medical personnel in mission hospitals and clinics around the world. Through its Post Residency program, WMM places post resident physicians in mission hospitals around the globe, where they serve two-year terms. They also staff a biomedical department and warehouse that provides critically needed medical equipment and supplies to medical mission facilities.

World Wide Lab - *www.wwlab.org*
A ministry that serves the laboratories in Christian mission hospitals and clinics in developing countries by providing affordable and durable equipment, supplies, training, and consulting.

Recommended Mission Conferences

Global Missions Health Conference – *www.medicalmissions.com*
A healthcare missions conference to inform, train, and equip healthcare professionals and students to use their skills to further God's kingdom. Co-sponsored by CMDA, this conference is usually held the second weekend in November at Southeast Christian Church in Louisville, Kentucky.

Orientation to Medical Missions – *www.cmda.org/orientation*
A conference hosted by CMDA's Center for Medical Missions which focuses on the unique challenges and opportunities in healthcare missions overseas. Preparing you to survive, thrive, and stay alive while serving in a cross-cultural setting. This is a small conference designed to offer personal contact and access to conference staff who have years of experience in career medical missions.

Training of Trainers Course –
www.lifewind.org or *www.equipministries.org*
A two-phase training course provided by LifeWind International or Equip International. The first phase is aimed at understanding the biblical basis for community health evangelism (CHE) and basic principles of wholistic community-based development. Participants learn basic skills for raising awareness, organizing, and mobilizing the community for cooperative action through the formation of a development committee. The second phase is designed to prepare trainers for two tasks: (1) equipping the development committee to lead the development process in their own community, and (2) training CHE volunteers for home visitation.

Recommended Mission Resources

Handbook of Medicine in Developing Countries - 3rd Edition
by Dennis Palmer, DO, and Catherine E. Wolf, MD
Medicine does not stand still in the U.S. or around the world. That is why CMDA published this third edition of *Handbook of Medicine in Developing Countries* which covers more diseases, has the latest treatment recommendations, includes sixteen pages of pictures of common dermatological diseases, and is easier to use than ever. If you are planning to go on a mission trip but have never worked overseas, this book is absolutely essential. Browse through it before you travel to prepare yourself for many of the common diseases and problems you will see. It will be as important to you as your airline tickets.

Medical Missions: Get Ready! Get Set! GO!
by Dr. Bruce Steffes
This book is the short-term medical mission GPS that will guide you every step of the way to successful service and ministry. It has chapters on reaching the unreached, picking an organization and planning your trip, raising support and building a support team, spiritual preparation, responding to the challenges of short-term medical missions, personal witnessing, other things one could do, education as a short-term missionary paradigm, reentry, "if only...", and I've come and gone, now what?

On Being A Missionary
by Thomas Hale, MD
This book was written for everyone who has an interest in missions, from the praying and giving supporter back home to the missionary on the field or about to be. It is not designed to be a theoretical textbook. It does not put forward new theses or new approaches to missions, nor does it attempt to break new ground. Instead, the author tries to absorb and then present the ideas, experiences, and insights of more than one hundred missionary writers. Drawing on his own years of experience, the author deals with problems, struggles, and failures of missionaries. It is from these that we learn the most. The goal is to ensure that when you get to the field you will be able to avoid many of the problems that have plagued others. Being a missionary is one of the most joyous and rewarding careers possible, and this book aims to make it ever more so.

Recommended Mission Resources

Operation World - 7th Edition
by Jason Mandryk
When you hear a country mentioned in the news or in a conversation and you want to know more about it and what God is doing there, this book will help you. Engage your heart and mind in global prayer with the thoroughly researched, fully updated seventh edition. It is loaded with clear, concise, and accurate information on peoples, languages, religions, denominations, spiritual trends, and prayer needs for every country in the world.

Preach and Heal: A Biblical Model for Missions
by Charles Fielding, MD
Can you imagine what would happen if we started mixing doctoring and church planting together? In the Gospel of Luke, Jesus sent His disciples to preach the kingdom of God and heal the sick. Jesus practiced both. *Preach and Heal* explores the ideology and practical ways for balanced ministry so that you can effectively reach the lost.

The Dental Handbook for Short-Term Mission Trips Booklet
by Global Health Outreach
This booklet begins with the GHO philosophy of care, dental treatment objectives, and clinical care guidelines for short-term mission trips. It includes many excellent checklists of dental instruments and supplies that will probably be needed on any mission trip you participate in. Besides providing material lists, there are also suggested protocols and other information that you will find helpful, particularly if you've never been on a mission trip before. If you have been on trips before, there are several pages concerning the responsibilities of the trip's dental director. Whether you are experienced in missions or not, this handy booklet will help you be prepared to serve those with desperate needs.

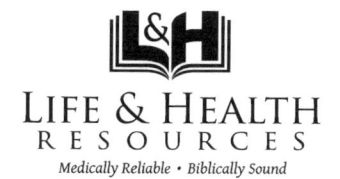

LIFE & HEALTH RESOURCES
Medically Reliable • Biblically Sound

More books on missions, cross-cultural issues, and biographies are available at *www.shopcmda.org*.

PHOTO GALLERY

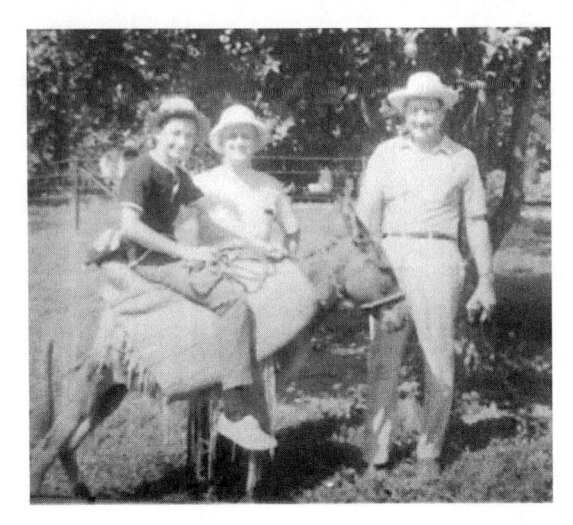

A teenage David Stevens rides a donkey on his first mission trip to Haiti in 1966.

After spending a summer working with Dr. Ernie Steury at Tenwek Hospital in Kenya, David returned to the United States to finish medical school.

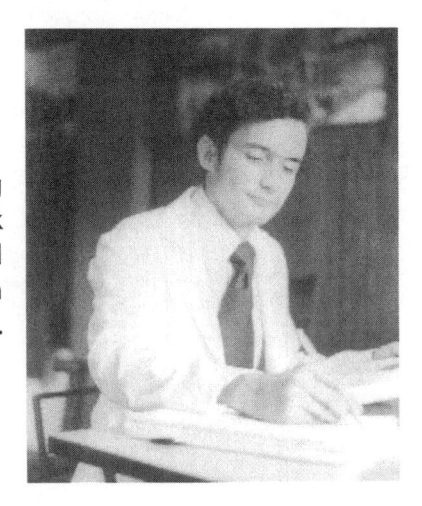

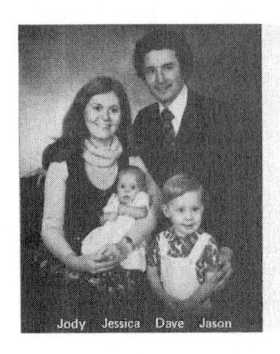

Along with his wife Jody and two children, the young family raised support to move to Kenya with this first prayer card in 1981.

Photo Gallery 337

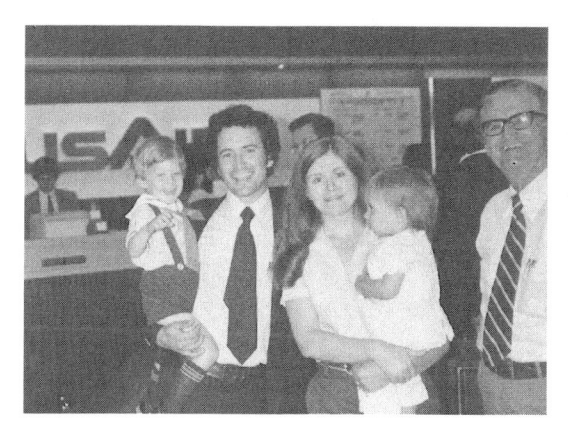

David, Jody, Jason and Jessica say goodbye to David's father Maurice Stevens at the airport before leaving for Kenya in 1981.

David and Jody study the Kipsigis language in 1981.

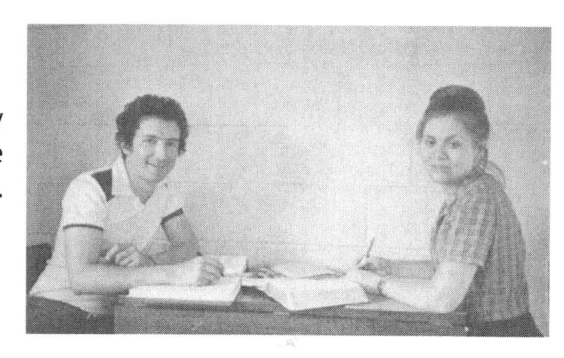

Jason and Jessica enjoying playtime with a few new friends and meet new baby sister Stacy, delivered by Dave in 1984.

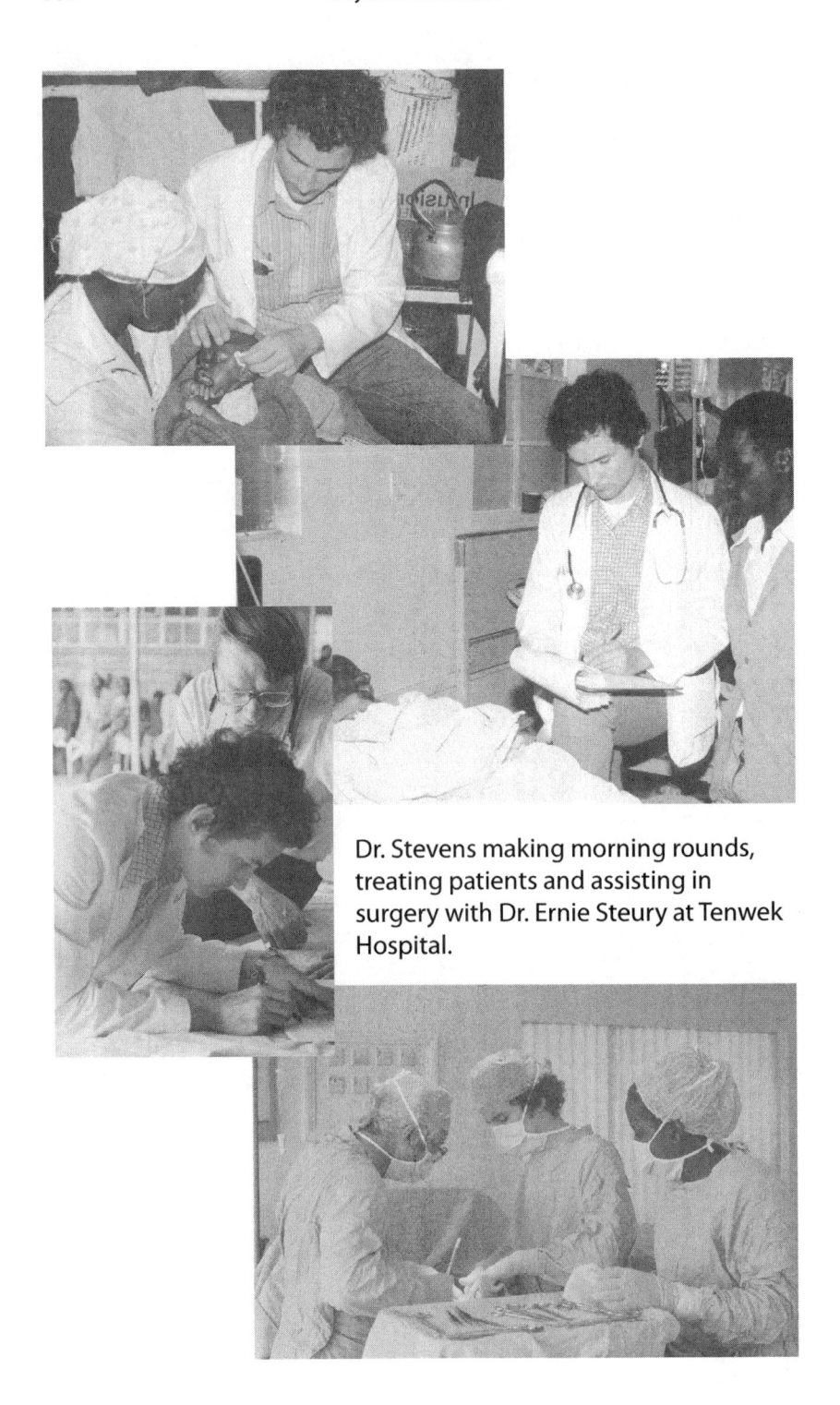

Dr. Stevens making morning rounds, treating patients and assisting in surgery with Dr. Ernie Steury at Tenwek Hospital.

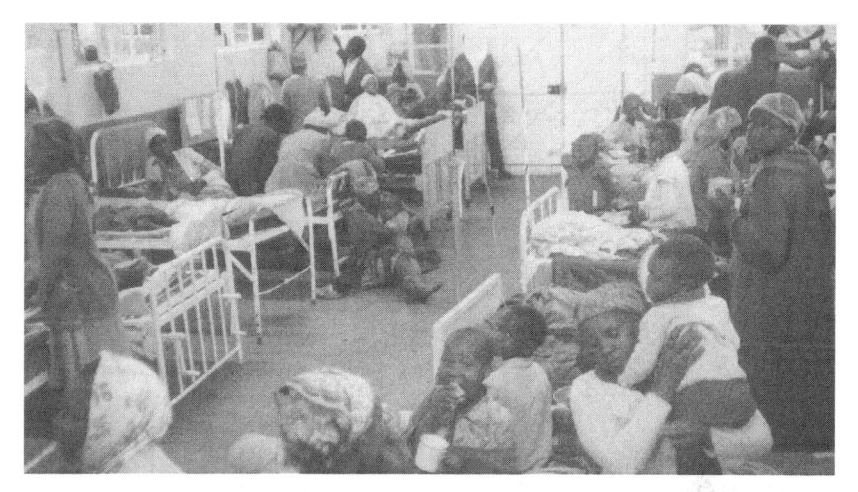

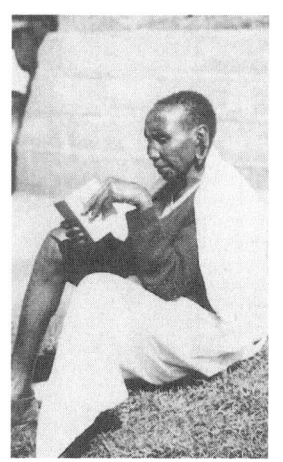

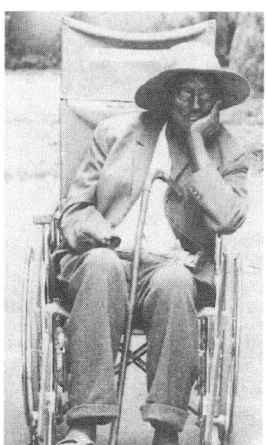

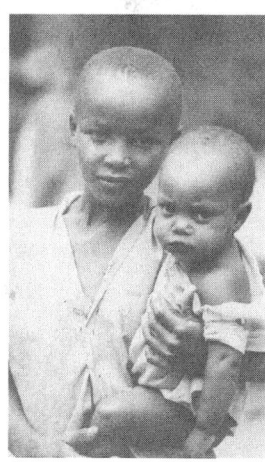

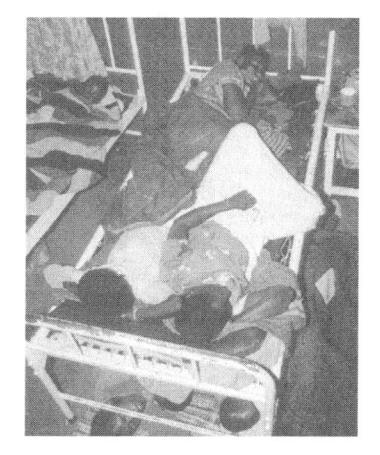

A few of the patients being treated at Tenwek Hospital.

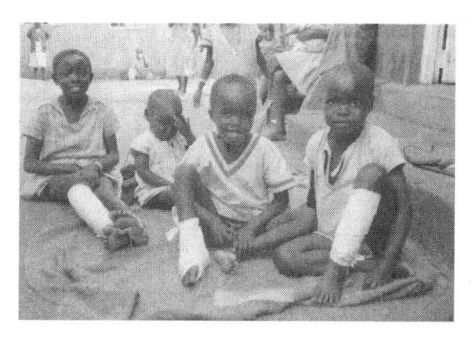

Enjoying family time amidst the busy and demanding schedules of being medical missionaries.

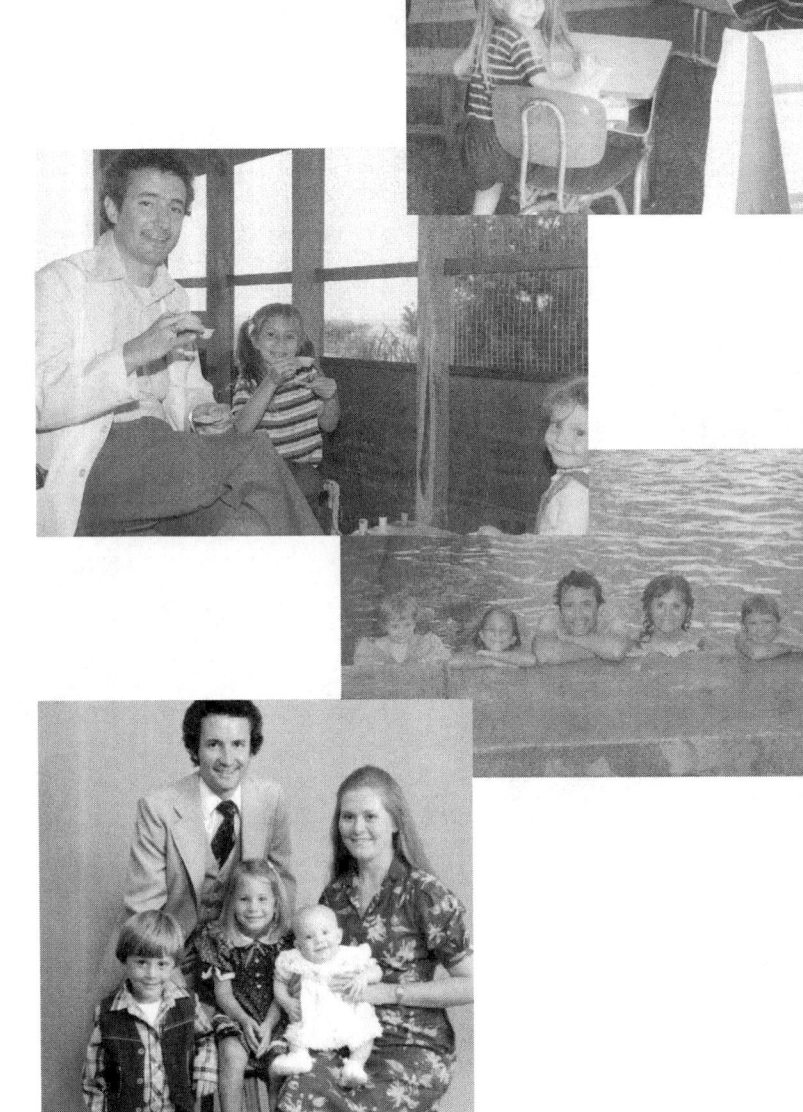

Photo Gallery 341

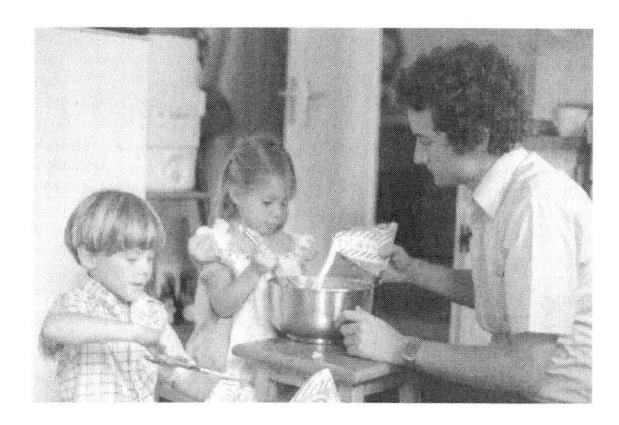

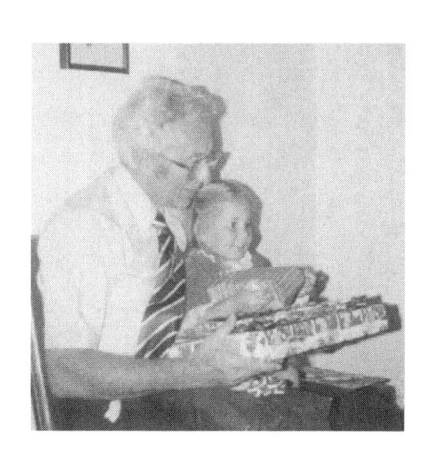

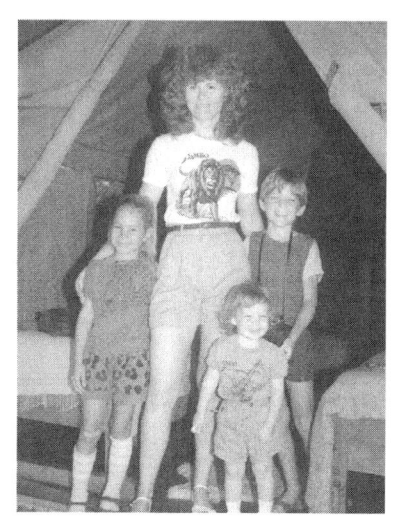

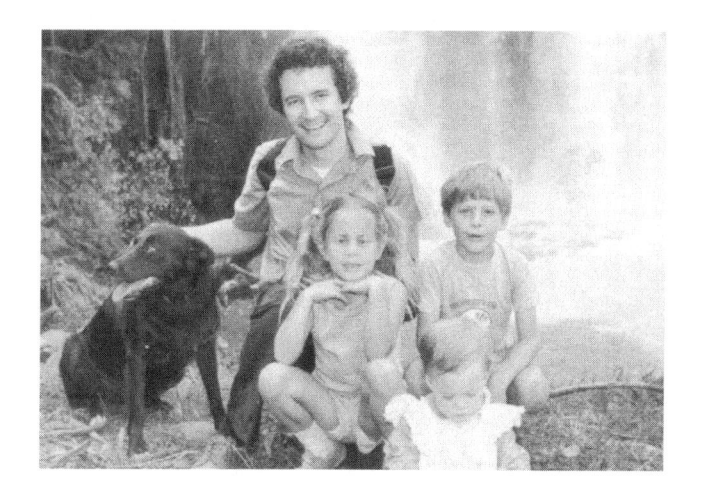

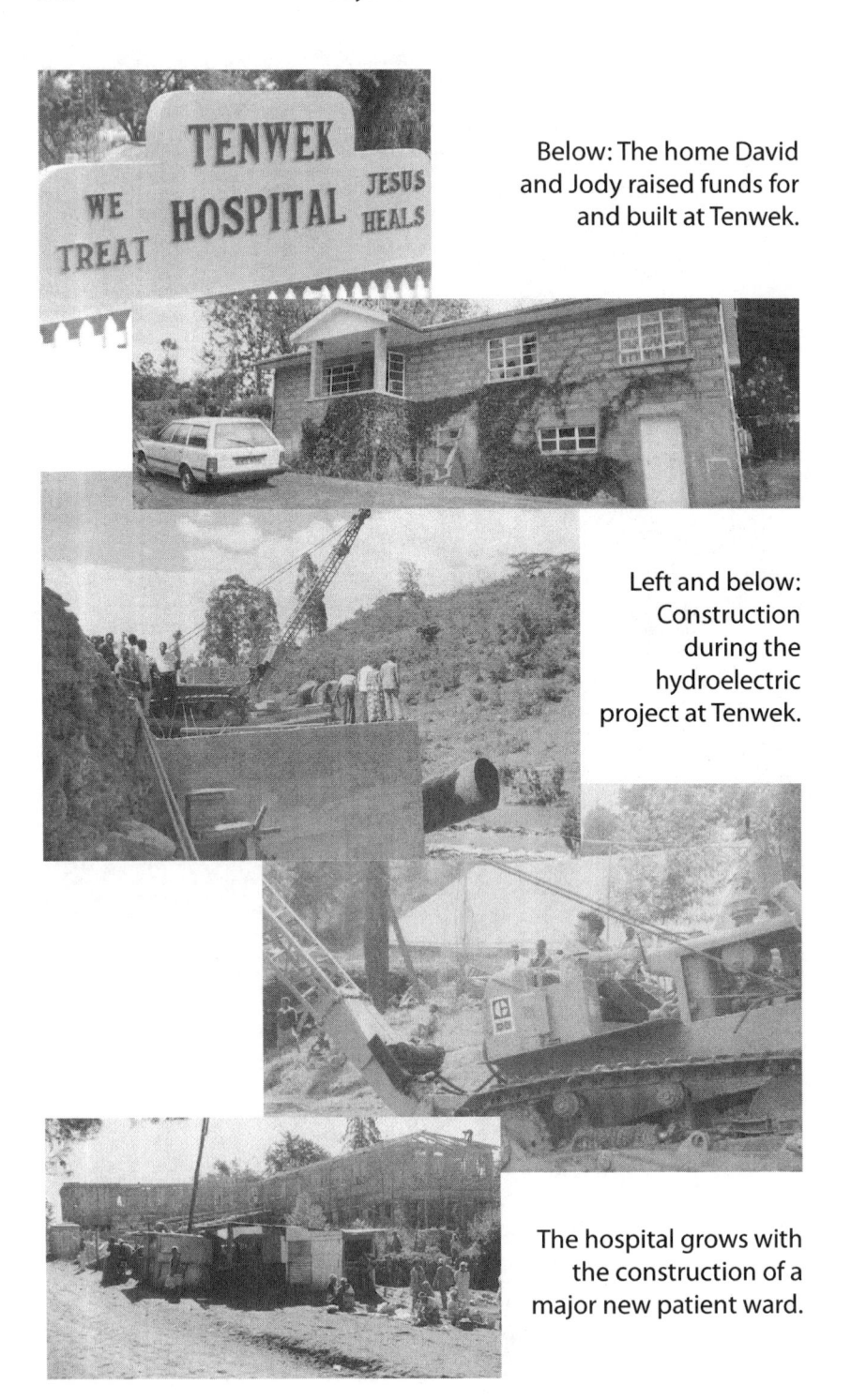

Below: The home David and Jody raised funds for and built at Tenwek.

Left and below: Construction during the hydroelectric project at Tenwek.

The hospital grows with the construction of a major new patient ward.

Photo Gallery

Susan Carter and Dr. Stevens direct the community health program.

A community health supervisor prepares to travel and meet with community health volunteers.

The first graduates from the community health program.

Dr. Stevens preaches during a district meeting.

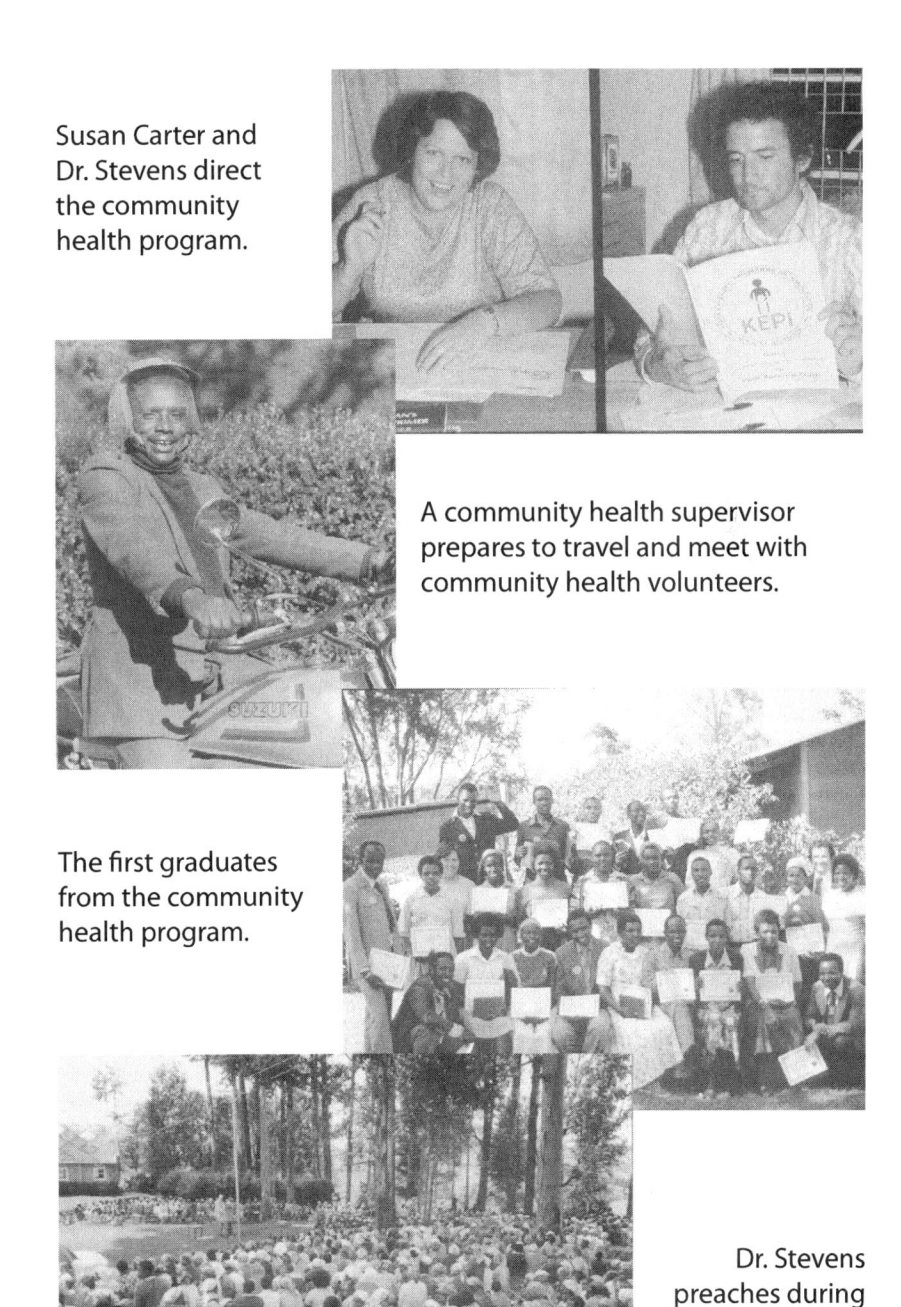

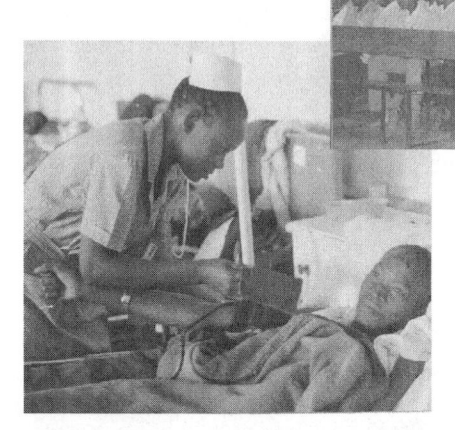

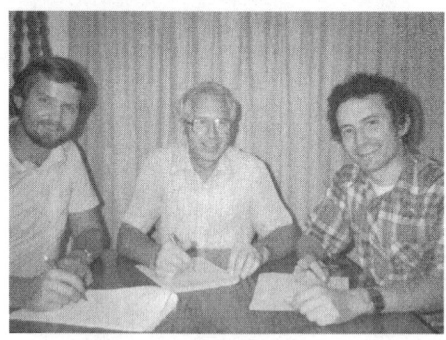

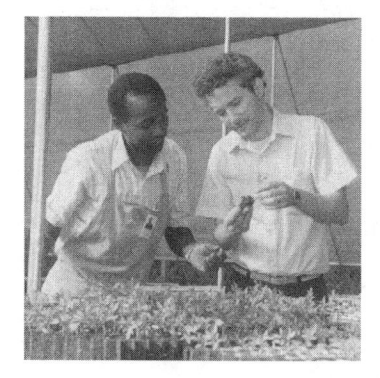

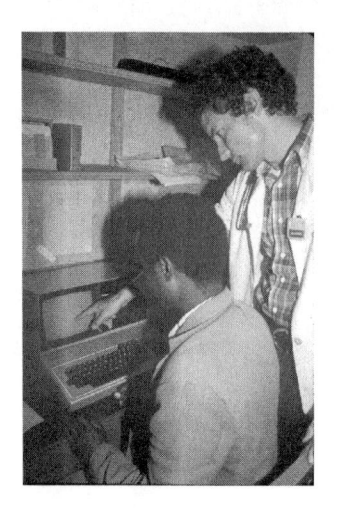

Other programs at Tenwek including the nursing program, agriculture development, computer training and pastoral training.

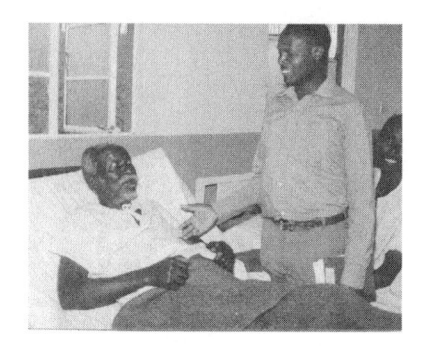

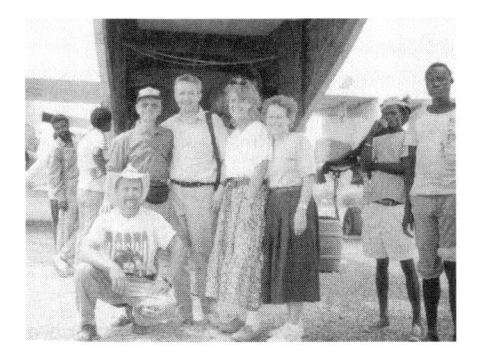

Dr. Stevens traveling to Bosnia, Somalia and Sudan to provide medical relief as the Director of World Medical Mission.

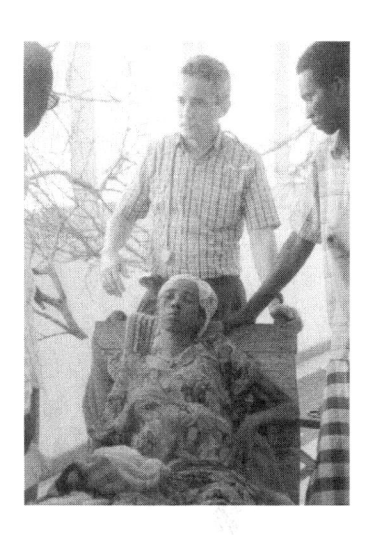

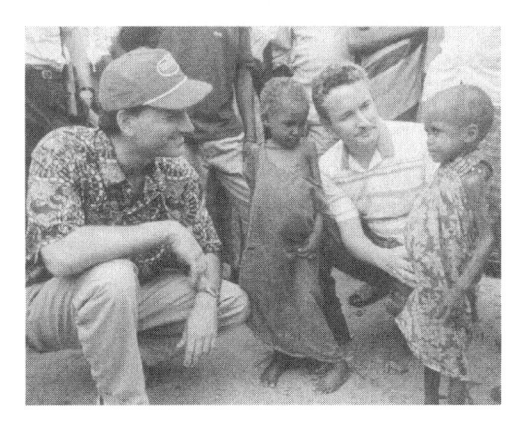

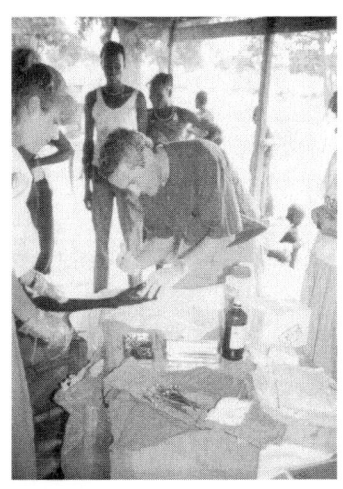

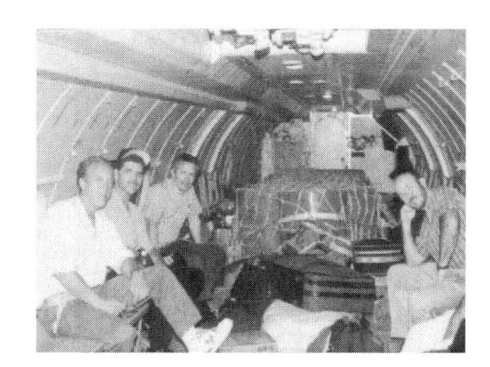